OXFORD MEDICAL PUBLICATIONS

Blood Disorders

THE FACTS

Blood Disorders

THE FACTS

SHEILA T. CALLENDER

Formerly Clinical Reader in Medicine,
John Radcliffe Hospital,
Oxford

OXFORD   NEW YORK   TOKYO
OXFORD   UNIVERSITY   PRESS
1985

Oxford University Press, Walton Street, Oxford OX2 6DP

Oxford New York Toronto
Delhi Bombay Calcutta Madras Karachi
Kuala Lumpur Singapore Hong Kong Tokyo
Nairobi Dar es Salaam Cape Town
Melbourne Auckland

and associated companies in
Beirut Berlin Ibadan Nicosia

Oxford is a trade mark of Oxford University Press

Published in the United States
by Oxford University Press, New York

British Library Cataloguing in Publication Data

Callender, Sheila T.
Blood disorders: the facts.
1. Blood——Diseases
I. Title
616.1'5   RC636
ISBN 0-19-261473-8

Library of Congress Cataloging in Publication Data

Callender, Sheila T.
Blood disorders.

(Oxford medical publications)
Includes index.
1. Blood——Diseases. I. Title. II. Series.
[DNLM: 1. Hematologic Diseases. WH 100 C157b]
RC636.C35   1985   616.1'5   85-15294
ISBN 0-19-261473-8

Typeset by Colset Private Limited, Singapore
Printed in Great Britain by R. Clay & Co. Ltd.,
Bungay, Suffolk

Preface

Unlike many of the other books in this series this one does not deal with a single disease but with a great variety of disorders which have in common only the fact that they are characterized by abnormalities in the blood. Virtually any illness may cause alterations in the blood, often enabling a diagnosis to be made on examination of the blood alone. The present volume, however, deals mainly with primary disorders of the blood rather than those secondary to other diseases, but the dividing line is often indistinct.

The aim has been to give some understanding of the functions of the various components of the blood, and to outline some of the disorders arising from disturbances in normal function. Many patients are bewildered by the apparently irrelevant investigations which may be needed to find the cause of a particular blood disorder, and I hope this book may help to enlighten them by indicating the reasons behind such tests.

There is a great variation in incidence of different blood disorders throughout the world. Some variation depends on economic conditions, social traditions and interaction with other diseases, but shifting populations and immigrations have played an important role over the centuries in changing the prevalence of some of the genetic disorders of the blood. This has been evident in Britain over the last decades with the increase in peoples of Cypriot, West Indian, and Asian origin, and has warranted the inclusion of blood disorders which were unfamiliar in this country a few years ago.

Fifty years ago very few of the disorders described here were treatable. To many a diagnosis was a death sentence, and many physicians felt it right to conceal the truth. This has

Preface

changed; many people with diseases which used to be fatal, now lead normal and active lives as a result of dramatic advances in treatment. The necessity to ensure cooperation in complicated regimes of treatment has resulted in a more open approach with benefit to both patient and doctor. Nevertheless confusions sometimes arise and it is hoped that this book may help with further understanding.

I acknowledge with gratitude the encouragement of Professor D.J. Weatherall and his help and that of Dr Elizabeth Gore in reading the manuscript and making useful suggestions. I am indebted to several colleagues for providing me with material for some of the illustrations, and to Blackwell Scientific Publications for permission to reproduce others. Special thanks are due to Mr John Hobbs for processing some of the photographs and to Mrs Janet Watt for her patience and expertise in typing the manuscript.

Oxford   S.T.C.
April 1985

Contents

To my former patients

1

Blood cells and their life story

When blood is put into a bottle, mixed with a substance which prevents clotting, it settles into various layers. At the top is a clear yellowish fluid, the 'plasma'; at the bottom a mass of red cells, and between a narrow whitish layer, which consists of the white cells and platelets. The total volume of blood in the body is normally about 4–5 litres. The blood plasma makes up about 55 per cent of this. Over 90 per cent of the plasma is water in which various fats, salts, sugars, vitamins, enzymes, and hormones are dissolved or suspended. Some 7 per cent is made up of proteins including those concerned with clotting of blood and others responsible for immunity to disease (immunoglobulins). Serum is the term used in place of plasma for the altered fluid resulting from the clotting of blood.

The red cells

The red cells (or erythrocytes) make up about 45 per cent of the total blood volume, and there are normally about 4–5 million in every cubic millimetre of blood; a drop about the size of a pin head. Unlike most cells in the body which have two main components, the nucleus which contains all the genetic material and a surrounding area called the cytoplasm, the red blood cells of all mammals have normally lost their nuclei by the time they enter the circulation. Those of all other vertebrates retain a nucleus.

Human red cells are shaped like tiny biconcave discs of fairly uniform size, measuring about 7.2 thousandths of a millimetre in diameter (Fig. 1). An important feature is their flexibility which allows them to squeeze through the narrowest of tiny blood-vessels, the capillaries, connecting the smaller arteries and veins. As will be seen later, abnormalities in the

Blood Disorders

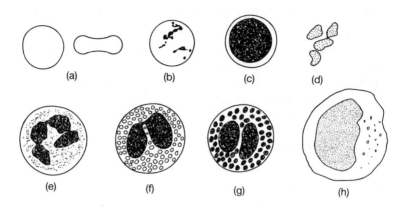

Fig. 1. Cells found in the blood; approximate relative size (a) red cells showing biconcave disc shape; (b) young red cell (reticulocyte); (c) lymphocyte; (d) platelets; (e) neutrophil granulocyte; (f) Eosinophil granulocyte; (g) basophil granulocyte; (h) monocyte.

shape or flexibility of the red cells are important facets of some blood disorders.

The membrane or envelope of the red cell was thought at one time to be a kind of inert bag, but it is now known to have a very complex structure. The membrane is responsible for maintaining the shape of the red cell. It also has a system which controls the concentrations of the elements sodium and potassium within the cell. This system requires energy which is provided by enzymes. Blood group markers such as ABO and Rh (rhesus) are attached to the membrane.

The principal function of the red cell is to carry oxygen, which it picks up as it passes through the small blood-vessels in the lungs, and delivers to the tissues throughout the body. There it is exchanged for carbon dioxide which in turn is returned to the lungs to be got rid of in the breath. This transport of oxygen depends on a special substance, haemoglobin, which is the main constituent of the red cell and gives blood its red colour. Scientists know almost more about the structure and function of haemoglobin than any other

2

molecule. It is made up of a protein part, globin, and an iron-containing molecule, haem. The globin consists of two pairs of chains (peptide chains) made up of organic molecules called amino acids. The precise arrangement of the amino acids and completeness of the chains is essential to the normal function of haemoglobin. Even minute variations can give rise to serious disorders of function.

One iron-containing molecule (haem) is attached to each peptide chain, and it is the iron which is responsible for the uptake and release of oxygen. Oxygenated blood is bright red in colour, that returning from the tissues to the lungs through the veins has lost its oxygen and is dark red or bluish in colour.

The white cells

There are normally far fewer white cells or leucocytes than red cells in circulation; only some 4–5 thousand in every cubic millimetre. They are of three main types: granulocytes, monocytes and lymphocytes (Fig. 1). All are concerned with defence against infection.

The granulocytes are so called because they contain characteristic granules. In the majority the nucleus is divided into two to five lobes, and the granules are very fine and stain a light pink with the dyes used to stain blood films; these are the neutrophils. These cells are capable of squeezing between the cells lining the blood-vessels to make their way to sites of injury, infection, or inflammation to which they are attracted by special substances (called chemotactic agents) produced at such sites. The main function of the neutrophils is to ingest foreign material by the process of phagocytosis. They remove debris from injury or inflammation and engulf and digest bacteria. In response to bacterial infection the granulocyte output is increased, and the mass of white cells which congregates at the site of an infection forms pus.

Some 2–4 per cent of the granulocytes have a spectacle-shaped nucleus and large granules which stain orange-red with the dye eosin. These 'eosinophils' are associated particularly with allergic conditions and infestation with parasites, when they are often found to be greatly increased in numbers (eosinophilia). The exact function of the eosinophils is unknown.

The least common type of granulocyte is the 'basophil', which has large deep purple-staining granules containing a number of substances associated with severe allergic responses.

Monocytes are the largest of the white cells in the blood (Fig. 1). The nucleus has no lobes and the granules are faint and few in number. Like the granulocytes the monocytes are active phagocytes.

Lymphocytes (Fig. 1) represent between 20 and 45 per cent of the circulating white cells. They are mostly smaller than the other white cells with a nucleus that almost fills the cell. Recent research has shown that, although all lymphocytes are concerned with development of immunity, there are several subgroups all of which perform different functions. One subtype, 'B cells', when stimulated can be transformed into cells called 'plasma cells' whose function is to produce antibodies. These are special proteins (immunoglobulins) which can attack foreign cells or substances that may be harmful. The sites which they attack are called 'antigens'. The object is to neutralize the foreign body and make it harmless, as in the development of immunity to infection, but as will be seen later such reactions can sometimes be harmful rather than beneficial.

In early childhood, before the age of about 5 years, lymphocytes are more numerous than granulocytes, but after this age the proportions are gradually reversed.

Platelets or thrombocytes

The smallest cells in the blood are the platelets or thrombocytes. These are tiny granular particles which are essential for the control of bleeding. They stick together readily and so plug up the smallest damaged blood-vessels and adhere to any

injured lining of larger blood-vessels. There are about 150–400
thousand platelets in every tiny drop of blood.

The origin and life span of the blood cells

All the cells in the blood are descendants of primitive cells in
the bone marrow called 'stem cells'. The existence of such a
common ancestor has been shown by experimental work
involving culture of cells. Given the appropriate stimulus, the
stem cells change, by a process called differentiation, into
clearly recognizable immature forms of the various cell types.

The production of red cells is normally controlled by a
hormone, erythropoietin, which is produced mainly by the
kidneys. The output of erythropoietin is in turn controlled by
the oxygen supply to the tissues. If this is reduced more
erythropoietin is produced; on the other hand, an increase in
oxygen supply depresses erythropoietin output. Erythropoietin stimulates the primitive red cells (erythroblasts) which
each produce about sixteen daughter cells by successive
divisions. During the process of division the cells mature and
change in appearance. Two vitamins are essential for normal
maturation, vitamin B_{12} and folic acid. During the later stages
in the bone marrow haemoglobin develops in the cytoplasm of
the red cells, a step which requires iron. The total time spent in
the bone marrow is about 7 days.

Before release of the red cells into the circulation the nuclei
are expelled, but a small amount of nuclear material remains
in the cytoplasm which appears as dots or a fine network on
special staining. These young cells are called 'reticulocytes'
and the numbers which are released into the blood are an indication of the activity of the bone marrow, and are a useful
measurement both in diagnosis and in assessing the response
to treatment of anaemia. They normally represent only about
1 per cent of the circulating red cells (Fig. 1).

After release into the blood the red cells have a fairly
uniform life span of about 120 days. The wornout cells are

then removed from circulation by scavenging cells called reti-culoendothelial cells which are distributed widely throughout the tissues particularly in the spleen, liver, and bone marrow. During the destruction of the old red cells the haem and globin of haemoglobin are separated: the iron is split off from the haem and returned to the bone marrow to make new cells, the rest of the haem is broken down in the liver to form bile pigment. If the life span of the red cells is greatly reduced, as in some anaemias, and many cells are destroyed rapidly, the liver may not be able to process the pigment immediately. This causes a form of jaundice with characteristic yellowing of the whites of the eyes and the skin.

Normally the majority of the cells in the bone marrow are early forms of the granulocyte. The earliest recognizable ancestors of these cells are called myeloblasts. Like the erythroblasts they go through several cell divisions while maturing. In the later stages of maturation division is no longer possible, but the characteristic granules develop and the nucleus is reduced in size and becomes lobed. After release from the bone marrow granulocytes remain in the circulation for only a matter of hours and then they migrate to the tissues to fulfil their role of combating infection.

Monocyte precursors (monoblasts) are not normally recog-nizable in the marrow but there is good evidence that they originate there. After release from the bone marrow, they soon leave the blood and go to the tissues where some become fixed, especially in the spleen, liver, lymph nodes and marrow to form the reticuloendothelial system. The life span of some of the tissue monocytes may be as long as months or even years.

The bone marrow is also a major site of production of lymphocytes. Their earliest ancestors are called lymphoblasts but they are not easily distinguished from other cells in normal bone marrow. After release lymphocytes migrate to various areas of lymphoid tissue, the masses of lymphocytes which are found in the lymph glands, spleen, and walls of the intestines.

Blood cells and their life story

From these areas there is a continuous recirculation and many of the lymphoid cells may live for years.

Platelets are derived from large cells in the bone marrow called megakaryocytes. Tiny fragments of the cytoplasm of these cells separate and are released into the blood. These may survive for 8–10 days and are then removed by the reticulo-endothelial cells.

2

Tests for blood disorders

Examination of the blood

Since almost any illness produces changes in the blood, one of the first tests a doctor may require as an aid to diagnosis is a blood count. This is made on a sample of blood taken from a vein and added to an anticoagulant to prevent clotting. The widespread use of electronic counters makes measurement of the number of red cells, white cells, and platelets, and the level of haemoglobin a simple matter, and the results are more accurate than the more laborious manual methods. These results are expressed as the number of cells in a litre of blood. The haemoglobin is measured in grams per decilitre (g/dl). Another useful measurement is the proportion of red cells to plasma (the packed cell volume or PCV) from which the average size of the red cells and their content of haemoglobin can be calculated.

A thin smear of blood on a glass slide is stained to reveal the proportion of the different cell types and any variation from normal. This examination alone may give an immediate diagnosis and is the most important part of the blood examination.

In disease the red cells may be too few in number (anaemia) or too many (polycythaemia). They may vary widely in shape (poikilocytosis) or in size (anisocytosis). When smaller than normal they are described as microcytes, when larger macrocytes. They may be deficient in haemoglobin (hypochromia). Young red cells are often larger than average and show some bluish staining (polychromasia); such cells on special staining are shown up as reticulocytes. In some blood disorders a few immature red cells which still retain a nucleus, may escape into the blood from the bone marrow.

The white cells may be increased in number (leucocytosis) or reduced (leucopenia) and such changes may affect any of the cell types. For example, septic infections tend to produce an increase in the granulocyte cells, whereas virus infections produce changes in the lymphocytes. Primitive white cells which are normally confined to the bone marrow may be identified in the blood film in conditions such as leukaemia.

The platelets again may be reduced in number (thrombocytopenia) or increased above a normal number (thrombocytosis). The former changes may be severe enough to cause bleeding, the latter may encourage thrombosis.

Bone marrow examination

A blood examination alone may not always be sufficient to arrive at a diagnosis, but a sample of bone marrow may give valuable additional information.

In infancy active bone marrow is found throughout the skeleton, but by adult life most of it has been replaced by fat cells. However, areas of active blood formation persist in the ribs, sternum (breastbone), the vertebrae (backbone), pelvic bones, skull, and the ends nearest to the body of the long bones in both arms and legs. In response to anaemia, the bone marrow may re-expand to replace the fat.

Various sites may be used to sample bone marrow. In young children the upper part of the tibia (shinbone) is usually chosen. In older children and adults the choice is between the sternum, the pelvis, or one of the spines of the vertebrae. If carefully done, after the injection of a little local anaesthetic, the insertion of the needle is almost painless and there should be only a brief discomfort as a few drops of the red bone marrow are sucked out into a syringe. However, if a patient is very apprehensive, or has to undergo several marrow punctures for control of treatment, a mild sedative or a short-lasting intravenous anaesthetic can be used. The marrow is spread on a glass slide and stained like a blood film. Some may also be put into special preservatives for other tests.

Erythrocyte sedimentation rate (ESR)

Another common and useful blood investigation is the erythrocyte sedimentation rate (ESR). This measures the rate at which a column of blood settles in a standard tube over a period of an hour. It is expressed as millimetres per hour (mm/h), the value being the difference between the original level of the red cells and that reached as the red cells settle down the column through the plasma. An increase in the ESR is not specific to a particular disorder and occurs in many conditions, but very rapid sedimentation indicates a disturbance in the plasma proteins and may point the way to further investigations.

The tests indicated above are only the starting point for arriving at a diagnosis in blood disorders, but they may lead to more specific tests which are mentioned in the chapters which follow.

3

Inheritance and blood disorders

Several blood disorders are the result of inherited abnormalities, and to save repetition a brief summary of the meaning of some of the genetic terms used and types of inheritance follows.

Chromosomes

The nucleus of every human cell contains a bunch of tiny strands of material called chromosomes, each of which is made up of many units called genes. Each gene has its own place in a particular chromosome and is responsible for a particular characteristic, but it may have several alternative forms called 'alleles'. When genes for particular characteristics are sited close together on one chromosome they are inherited together and are said to be 'linked'. The combination of alleles in this situation is called a 'haplotype'.

Every cell, with the exception of the sperm cells and eggs, has 46 chromosomes (23 pairs) (Plate 1). Techniques have been devised for the recognition of the individual pairs of chromosomes which are released from the nucleus and replicate during cell division. Of these, 22 have been given numbers 1–22 and are called 'autosomes'. The 23rd pair are the sex chromosomes X and Y. The sexes are distinguished by females having two X chromosomes and males an X and a Y. The sperm and eggs have only half the number of chromosomes, one of each pair, during fertilization each parent, therefore, contributes half of each pair in the cells of the resulting embryo.

Blood Disorders

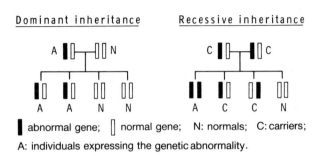

Fig. 2. Patterns of dominant and recessive autosomal inheritance.

Autosomal inheritance

Conditions which are determined by an abnormality of a gene on one of the autosomes are described as having 'autosomal inheritance'. If one of a pair of genes is abnormal and the other normal the individual is described as 'heterozygous' for the gene, or a 'heterozygote' or 'carrier'. If both genes of the pair have the same abnormality the individual is 'homozygous', or a 'homozygote' for the defect. Autosomal inheritance may be dominant or recessive (Fig. 2). If dominant both heterozygotes and homozygotes will show the defect. With recessive inheritance only those individuals acquiring the genetic abnormality from both parents — in other words, homozygotes — will show the disorder. In some blood conditions, although only the homozygotes have disabling disease, the heterozygotes or carriers of the abnormal gene have detectable changes in the blood, allowing recognition of the carrier state. This is sometimes referred to as intermediate inheritance rather than a true recessive inheritance.

Sex-linked inheritance

In 'sex-linked inheritance' the abnormality is carried on one of the sex chromosomes (Fig. 3). Haemophilia is a classic example of a blood disorder with X-linked inheritance.

Inheritance and blood disorders

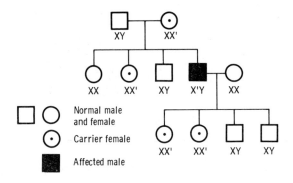

Fig. 3. An example of sex-linked inheritance (X^1 the abnormal gene).

Carrier females are normal due to the presence of a normal X chromosome as well as the defective one, but any sons who inherit her abnormal X chromosome will have haemophilia. There is an even chance of this happening and an even chance of her daughters being carriers. All daughters of an affected male will be carriers, but all *his* sons will be normal.

Chromosome abnormalities

In some blood conditions abnormalities of chromosomes are acquired, for example by breaks in the chromosomes or by bits of one chromosome being joined to one of the others (translocation). Some such abnormalities are so constant and characteristic as to become useful in diagnosis, for example the 'Philadelphia' chromosome which occurs in chronic myeloid leukaemia (see p. 114) and is the result of a translocation.

4

Symptoms and causes of anaemia

It is difficult to define the borderline between normal blood and anaemia. The World Health Organization, as a result of many studies, has defined anaemia in terms of the level of haemoglobin, taking a value of 13 grams per decilitre (g/dl) for men and 12 g/dl for women as the lower limit of normal. However, as in any biological measurement, there is considerable variation in values among normal healthy subjects, and an overlap between ranges of optimal and suboptimal haemoglobin values. With the latter the haemoglobin may be increased by appropriate treatment.

Symptoms of anaemia

It is generally supposed that any degree of anaemia gives rise to symptoms such as tiredness, headaches, palpitations, and breathlessness, but while such symptoms may certainly occur in association with anaemia they may equally be caused by stress, depression, or other illness. A fall in haemoglobin leads to lack of adequate oxygen supply to the tissues. The body can adapt to this by stepping up the production of red cells, but if for any reason this is not possible the rate of circulation of the blood can be increased and, more specifically, a red cell enzyme which enhances the efficiency with which oxgyen is delivered to the tissues may be increased. Because of these adaptations minor degrees of anaemia may produce little or no symptoms. Even in quite severe anaemia, provided that the condition has progressed very slowly, adaptation may be remarkably efficient and the patient may recognize the disability only by how much better he or she feels after effective treatment. On the other hand, a rapid onset of anaemia will be accompanied by far more serious symptoms. In the elderly, degenerative changes in blood-vessels may reduce the tolerance to anaemia and cause symptoms of angina or cardiac failure.

Causes of anaemia

World wide the commonest types of anaemia are due to malnutrition and infections. At one time this was the case in all poor communities, but in the developed world the picture has changed dramatically, especially over the last 50 years. Improvements in standards of living, better education and health care, and the advent of antibiotics have all played a role in reducing the incidence of both malnutrition and infections, thus changing the prevalence of many kinds of anaemia.

Anaemia may be caused in a variety of ways. There may be a failure of production of red cells with partial or complete absence of red cell formation in the bone marrow. In some conditions this is the result of replacement of normal bone marrow by other tissue such as a cancer or leukaemia. Other anaemias are due to lack of the building materials needed for normal development of red cells, such as vitamin B_{12}, folic acid, and iron. In yet others the red cells are destroyed more rapidly than normal, either because of an inherited defect in the cells or due to factors outside the red cell which result in their early death. These are called the haemolytic anaemias.

The distinction between the main groups of anaemia is not always clear cut since, for example, in many anaemias in which there is faulty production of cells, the cells which are produced also have a shortened life span.

5

Anaemia due to lack of building materials: (1) iron-deficiency

This type of anaemia will be described first since, apart from anaemias secondary to conditions such as chronic infections and malignancy, it is by far the commonest type. It is a world-wide problem in spite of the fact that iron is one of the most ubiquitous metals. In nature, however, iron exists largely in poorly available forms, and both plants and animals are prone to develop iron deficiency.

The prevalence of iron deficiency

In humans iron is an essential component of haemoglobin and it is also present in the protein of muscle, myoglobin. In addition, many enzymes involved in oxygen supply to the tissues contain iron. In the ideal state there should be sufficient iron available for an optimal haemoglobin and other normal requirements, plus some in storage to cover increased demands, for example following a haemorrhage.

Surveys made throughout the world have indicated that anaemia is a very common problem. The exact prevalence of iron deficiency is, however, difficult to establish particularly in countries where methods of investigation are limited, and other factors such as infections, general malnutrition, and abnormalities of haemoglobin structure play a significant role. Furthermore, many surveys are confined to selected groups of populations. In all countries, however, it is clear that iron deficiency affects mainly children, and women during their reproductive life.

Some telling studies were made in the early 1930s among the poorest classes in Aberdeen and north-east Scotland. The

Anaemia due to iron-deficiency

people studied were not selected because of ill-health, nevertheless 70 per cent of the pregnant women, almost half the younger women who had borne children, rather fewer (36 per cent) of child bearing women over the age of 45 and 25 per cent of women who had never borne children were anaemic, as were a high proportion of infants under the age of two. Anaemia was rare in men. These figures took no account of additional individuals with latent iron deficiency — a state where iron stores are exhausted but anaemia is not yet apparent.

As I know from my own experiences as a medical student, in the conditions at that time of gross poverty and overcrowding, many women existed on bread and cups of tea while their menfolk, whose needs for iron were far less, had the best of the scant food available. There was much ignorance about contraception and a dozen or more pregnancies were not uncommon. Back-street abortions resulted in gross blood loss. Some of the inadequate dole money was spent on Friday nights on such abortions, and women arrived at the hospital exanguinated. All that could be done was to curette the womb to stop the bleeding. Occasionally a single pint of blood might be available to resuscitate the patient, but the blood transfusion services that we now accept so readily were nonexistent.

This has all changed in western countries. Improvements in nutrition, better access to medical care, particularly child welfare and antenatal care, limitations to family size, and reduction of menstrual blood loss with the widespread use of the contraceptive pill, have all helped to reduce the incidence of iron deficiency, but still some 10–15 per cent of women of reproductive age suffer from iron-deficiency anaemia and at least as many again may have latent iron deficiency (Fig. 4). In many parts of the third world iron lack remains a major problem, often with anaemia of a severity seldom now seen in the more developed countries. In order to understand the causes of iron deficiency and the reasons why it is so common

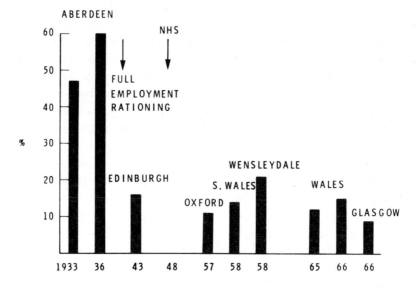

Fig. 4. The incidence of iron-deficiency anaemia in women, as reported in several surveys in the United Kingdom.

it is necessary to look at the balance between demand and supply of iron.

Iron requirements

The total amount of iron in a normal adult man is about 4 g. About three-quarters of this is accounted for by iron in the haemoglobin of circulating red cells, about 10 per cent is in myoglobin in muscles, and most of the remainder is found in the iron stores in the liver, spleen and bone marrow. The iron-containing enzymes account for a few milligrams (mg), and some is constantly in transport from one site to another attached to a special carrier protein in the plasma called transferrin.

Because of the continual reuse of the iron released from wornout red cells, the amount lost from the body each day is

18

very small. However, all cells contain traces of iron, and some are constantly being shed from the skin, the lining of the gut, and from the urinary tract. There are also traces of iron in the bile. This daily loss amounts to a total of less than 1 mg in the healthy adult man, and is all that he needs to replace from his diet. This, however, is the *minimum* iron requirement. The need varies greatly at different ages and between the sexes, and in some circumstances is far more than this basic amount.

A baby is born with a supply of iron obtained from the mother through the placenta (the afterbirth). It is remarkable that the baby's need has priority over that of the mother, so that even if she is short of iron, any released from her worn-out red cells goes to the fetus at her expense. This build-up of iron in the fetus occurs mainly in the last 3 months of pregnancy when the requirement may reach as much as 6 mg per day, or more with a multiple pregnancy. This has two effects; first, the mother is most likely to become iron-deficient in the last half of pregnancy; and second, if the baby is born prematurely it will not have had time to obtain the full amount of iron from its mother. Another factor which influences the amount of iron the child has at birth is the time at which the umbilical cord is tied. If this is too soon the baby may be deprived of a significant amount of iron in the form of blood from the placenta.

At birth a baby's haemoglobin is normally much higher than in later life. the excess red cells are destroyed in the early post natal weeks, and the iron freed in this way is added to the stores to help tide over a period of low iron intake from just milk alone.

As the baby grows there is an increase in blood volume and in muscle mass, both of which use up iron, so that by about 6 months of age the stores may be exhausted and the infant becomes prone to develop iron-deficiency anaemia if milk feeding alone goes on too long. If, however, mixed feeding is introduced, particularly with infant cereals which are usually supplemented with iron and vitamin C, iron deficiency can be prevented.

The next stage at which iron demand may overtake iron supply is during the growth spurt of puberty. When this is ended the iron requirement of a boy drops to that of an adult man, less than 1 mg per day, but in girls the onset of menstruation increases the iron need. Each month, on average, a woman loses about 30–40 ml of blood, the equivalent of about 15–20 mg of iron, and this represents an average extra requirement of about 0.5 mg of iron daily to make good the loss. About 10 per cent of women lose far more than this, and many do not recognize that their blood loss is abnormal, even though they may lose five to ten times the average. The upper limit beyond which iron deficiency is likely to develop is only 80 ml per menstrual period — rather less than half a tea cupful.

Pads and tampons for sanitary protection vary very considerably in their efficiency in absorbing blood, so that the number used per period is only a very rough guide to the amount of blood lost. As a general rule, women who can manage with internal tampons only probably do not lose excessive blood.

Pregnancy clearly increases the demand for iron (Fig. 5). Although there is no blood loss from menstruation the mother needs iron for the baby, the placenta and blood loss at delivery. In addition, the mother's red cell mass increases during pregnancy, and for this extra iron is temporarily needed. After delivery the red cell mass returns to normal and this iron is therefore conserved. Nevertheless, if the pregnancy has been started at a time when iron stores are low, the increase in red cell mass will increase the amount of iron needed from the diet. The total extra iron needed for a pregnancy is of the order of 1000 mg, but this is not evenly distributed throughout pregnancy. The increased need is from about the fourth month onwards and reaches a maximum during the last trimester. Lactation uses about the same amount of iron as

Anaemia due to iron-deficiency

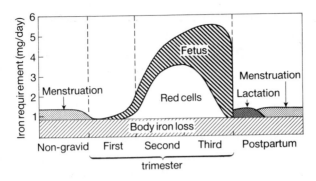

Fig. 5. The daily iron requirement for a normal pregnancy; in the first few weeks the need for iron may be reduced because menstruation has stopped, but during the second and third trimester the requirement increases steadily. (Courtesy of Professor T.H. Bothwell and Blackwell Scientific Publications.)

normal menstruation, in other words, about 0.5 mg per day.

In summary, iron needs are minimal in the normal adult man and post-menopausal woman, but they are increased during periods of rapid growth and in women during the reproductive years because of menstrual losses and the iron demands for pregnancy.

In addition to these physiological variations in iron requirement, clearly any cause of abnormal bleeding will increase the need for iron. This usually means a source of bleeding from the stomach or bowels such as may be caused by ulcers or piles. Some drugs, for example aspirin, may also cause internal bleeding in some people.

In tropical countries infestations of parasites are a common cause of blood loss, particularly hookworm infestation. One type of hookworm is also found in more temperate climates such as southern Europe and the Middle East. The larvae of the parasites enter the skin through the bare feet of people working in infected soil, and migrate to the walls of the intestine where they attach themselves to the lining. Each of these minute worms can suck about 0.1–0.25 ml of blood a

21

day. The load of worms is very variable but may amount to many thousands, enough to lead to very significant losses of blood. The higher the load the more likely it is that anaemia will develop.

Iron and nutrition

An average western type of diet (without supplementation) contains some 6 mg of iron per 1000 calories giving an intake of about 12–15 mg of iron per day. This assumes, of course, a daily calorie intake of about 2000–2500, whereas many figure-conscious young women may restrict their intake to nearer 1000 calories. Even at this lower daily intake, however, if all the iron could be absorbed people would suffer from the toxic effects of iron overload rather than iron shortage, but for various reasons a high proportion of iron in food is not available for absorption.

There are two main forms in which iron is present in food: as inorganic or non-haem iron compounds, which are the only source in vegetarian diets; and as haem compounds derived from muscle and haemoglobin in foods of animal origin. It is important to distinguish between the two types of dietary iron as they are dealt with differently during the processes of digestion and absorption.

The inorganic iron compounds in food are very readily influenced by interaction with other factors in the diet, and by the presence or absence of normal digestive secretions. In the stomach some of the iron is released during digestion, and is held in solution if the gastric juice is sufficiently acid, but after passing out of the stomach the iron meets the alkaline juices of the small intestine. In these conditions the iron comes out of solution (precipitates) and is less available for absorption. This is counteracted to some extent by the presence of other compounds in the gastric juice called mucoproteins and certain substances in the diet, particularly ascorbic acid (vitamin C) but also some sugars and alcohol, which form soluble complexes with iron. On the other hand, other factors in food — such as phytates and phosphates which are present in cereals, phosphoproteins in eggs, and the tannins in tea — form insoluble complexes with iron so reducing iron absorption. The proportion of non-haem iron reaching the absorptive cell surface of the duodenum and jejunum depends, therefore, on a great many interactions between the iron and the digestive secretions and other constituents in the food.

Haem iron is dealt with in an entirely different way. During digestion it is separated from the protein to which it has been attached, and after it passes into the intestine from the stomach it is absorbed as haem and the iron is not split off until the haem is inside the mucosal cells lining the intestine. Haem iron is therefore protected from the influence of the factors which alter absorption of the inorganic or non-haem iron.

The cells lining the small intestine are potentially capable of absorbing iron throughout the length of the small gut, but shortly beyond the first part (the duodenum and upper part of the jejunum) the alkaline conditions render this impossible, except for the haem iron. Thus damage to the upper part of the intestine from any cause reduces the absorption of non-haem iron.

Although for the reasons indicated above the available iron in the diet is very variable in amount, the ultimate control of absorption lies in the cells lining the intestine. How precisely this control is organized is not clear, but normally if the body has sufficient iron for its needs the cells hold on to most of the iron and do not pass it on into the blood. The unwanted iron is then lost when the cells are shed from the gut lining. If, however, there is an iron lack more iron is transported through the cells and so into the circulation where it becomes attached to the carrier protein, transferrin. Most of this absorbed iron will be transported to the bone marrow. Any surplus to blood requirements will go to the stores.

Blood Disorders

Table 1

The average (mean) absorption of iron in normal and iron deficient subjects measured with the use of tracer doses of radioactive iron incorporated into various foods and compared with the absorption from a simple iron salt.

	Mean per cent of iron absorbed	
	Normal	Iron-deficient
Ferrous iron (5 mg)	9.2	40.1
White bread	2.2	7.3
Oat cakes and porridge	4.0	10.0
Eggs	2.2	5.6
Chicken	6.9	17.0
Haemoglobin	10.0	22.0

Iron deficiency can result in about a two to three-fold increase in iron absorption (Table 1), but if the availability of the iron in the diet is low this may make little absolute difference. People with iron deficiency may absorb some 20 per cent of the iron from a well-balanced diet containing iron of high availability, but the same individuals on a diet with the same iron content but in poorly available form may absorb less than 5 per cent, a difference perhaps between 3 mg and less than 1 mg, which is very significant when considered in the light of the iron requirements.

An increase in iron absorption may compensate partially for periods of increased need, but there comes a time at which supply cannot meet the demand. The iron in storage is then called upon and for a time this may be sufficient to prevent anaemia. Once the stores are gone, however, continued increased demands for iron will result in anaemia.

Much of what has been learnt about the complexities of

Anaemia due to iron-deficiency

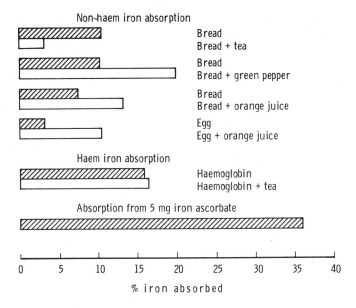

Fig. 6. Iron absorption from foods labelled with tracer amounts of radioactive iron; each pair of columns represents the mean per cent absorption in a group of iron-deficient patients.

absorption of iron from food has been made possible by the use of 'tracers' of radioactive iron. These are measurable but harmless amounts of radioactivity which can be used to 'label' different forms of iron or different foods.

In the examples illustrated in Fig. 6 the absorption of iron from some foods, and the effects of varying the constituents of a meal, are shown and compared with the absorption from a similar amount of iron in the form of a simple ferrous iron salt. The observations were made in iron-deficient people who showed a relatively high absorption of iron, but in all cases the iron was less well absorbed from food than from the iron salt. As can be seen, the absorption of non-haem iron is adversely affected by the addition of tea (due to tannin), but enhanced by orange juice and green peppers (both good sources of vitamin C). In contrast haem iron is relatively well absorbed and is not affected by the addition of tea.

Varying the constituents of the diet without altering the total iron content can clearly make a great difference to the amount available for absorption and the introduction of free orange juice and rose-hip syrup for pregnant women and children during the Second World War probably played a significant role in reducing the incidence of iron deficiency at that time because of the high vitamin C content of these supplements.

The clinical problem

While it is debatable how far general symptoms may be attributed to minor degrees of iron deficiency, a suboptimal haemoglobin, and lack of iron stores puts an individual at risk for developing more severe anaemia. There is also evidence that the capacity for physical work is reduced. More severe degrees of deficiency are accompanied by symptoms common to any anaemia, such as pallor, breathlessness on exertion, increased pulse rate and, when the haemoglobin reaches very low levels, swelling of the feet, ringing in the ears and anginal pain.

The more specific features of iron deficiency are conditioned by abnormalities in the iron-dependent enzymes. These features are not always present but are very characteristic when they are. The tongue is often glazed and painful (glossitis), and there may be soreness and cracks at the corners of the mouth (angular stomatitis). The latter is usually associated with poorly fitting dentures, or lack of teeth, and may be complicated by thrush infection. Another frequent complaint is of brittle nails. In long-standing iron deficiency this may progress to the development of deformed spoon-shaped nails (koilonychia (Plate 2)). These are seen less frequently than some years ago, possibly because women no longer spend hours at a wash-tub or scrubbing floors, their hands and nails exposed to the additional damaging effects of hot water and chemicals such as washing soda.

Occasionally, especially in older patients, there may be a complaint of difficulty in swallowing. This is associated with the formation of a web of tissue which partially obstructs the upper end of the food passage. It is felt typically just below the level of the Adam's apple. In a few instances it may go on to a more severe narrowing which requires dilatation. There is an increased risk of cancer developing at the site of such an obstruction.

Patients suffering from iron deficiency often have changes in the lining of the stomach (gastritis) resulting in partial or total loss of acid secretion. Although normally the secretion of gastric acid tends to be reduced with age, patients with iron deficiency are twice as likely to lack acid secretion (achlorhydria). It is not clear how far this is directly due to iron deficiency, but once established it is certainly a contributory factor to poor iron absorption.

Some individuals with iron deficiency develop a distorted appetite (pica) for substances such as paper, ice, or clay. This may in some cases be a consequence of the iron deficiency, but observations on clay eaters in southern Turkey have shown clearly that the particular clay in that locality can prevent iron absorption, and the pica there is therefore a cause rather than the result of iron lack.

The diagnosis of iron deficiency depends on a few simple tests. Various stages can be distinguished. In the earlier stages the body is depleted of iron, but there is still sufficient for the production of normal red cells, and the blood count will be normal. However, if the bone marrow is examined and stained for iron, none will be found in the storage cells (reticuloendothelial cells) which normally contain some iron.

Examination of the serum will show a reduced level of transferrin-bound iron, although the amount of the carrier protein transferrin is increased. Another protein, ferritin, which contains iron and is part of the pool of storage iron, can also be measured in the serum. In iron deficiency it is much reduced.

When the stores are depleted but iron needs remain high the condition changes from one of latent to overt iron deficiency with reduction in haemoglobin production. The red cells which are produced are small and misshapen and deficient in haemoglobin (hypochromic). This is easily recognized by the blood count and examination of the blood film (Plate 3).

However, to put a label to the blood findings does not establish a proper diagnosis, that depends on finding out why the deficiency of iron has arisen. There are three groups of causes which have to be considered; dietary deficiency, increased need and malabsorption of iron.

Dietary deficiency

Pure nutritional deficiency where the available iron in the diet is insufficient to meet normal physiological needs is rare except in children where milk feeding without any supplement has gone on too long. Poor diet may, however, contribute to the development of iron deficiency, particularly where through ignorance or poverty the diet is restricted to foods from which iron is poorly absorbed such as cereals and eggs, or when prolonged cooking destroys the vitamin C in the food.

Increased need

An unusually high requirement for iron may be due to increased physiological need such as that due to heavy menstrual periods or multiple pregnancies, or to pathological blood loss from the gut or, much less frequently, from the urinary tract.

In women of reproductive age by far the commonest cause of iron deficiency is excessive menstrual loss. Sometimes a gynaecological examination shows the presence of a fibroid (a benign tumour arising in the wall of the womb), but in many women there is no detectable abnormality to account for the heavy loss.

In older women and men iron deficiency is likely to be due to blood loss from the gastrointestinal tract. Although, of course, in many cases there may be clear abdominal symptoms in others there may be nothing to point to the cause. Bleeding from piles, which is among the commonest causes of iron deficiency is obvious, but blood loss sufficient to lead to anaemia in other conditions may never have been noticed. One cause of bleeding which can easily be overlooked is aspirin, which can irritate the lining of the stomach and cause significant bleeding in some people.

It may need several different investigations to determine the cause of blood loss. Specimens of stool can be examined for traces of blood. X-rays of the stomach and bowel may be required. Sometimes a fibrescope (a flexible tube through which the inside of an organ can be examined) may need to be passed into the stomach or bowel to look for sites of bleeding.

If blood has been noted in the urine a whole range of kidney tests may be required including X-ray examinations.

Malabsorption of iron

Various gastrointestinal disorders may cause malabsorption of iron. As has already been mentioned, chronic gastritis with consequent loss of secretion of acid in the stomach will reduce absorption, but is unlikely to be the sole cause of iron deficiency. Stomach operations which involve bypass of the first part of the intestine, where iron is mainly absorbed, may also reduce absorption. In some such cases there is also a factor of more hurried transport of food past this area.

There is, however, a particular condition in which the absorption of iron is characteristically reduced. This is coeliac disease, a condition known to be caused by sensitivity of the lining of the upper part of the intestine to a protein in wheat, gluten. The condition is now often called 'gluten enteropathy'. The gluten damages the mucosal cells lining the gut and this lining, instead of presenting the normal frond-like appearance, becomes flattened affecting the absorption of a range of substances, among them iron. This condition is probably far more common than was previously realized and as many as one in 300 people in Britain may be affected, though often only to a minor degree. In the west of Ireland a familial incidence has been recognized.

In severe cases the clinical picture is dominated by the symptoms of fatty diarrhoea and the diagnosis is made in early childhood. Many people, however, reach adult life with little or no abdominal symptoms, and are diagnosed only because they have a chronic iron-deficiency anaemia which fails to respond to iron treatment. Because the upper part of the small intestine is damaged by gluten, only the absorption of non-haem or inorganic iron is affected; haem iron can still be absorbed further down the gut.

Delayed puberty or short stature, as compared with parents and siblings, may suggest the diagnosis of coeliac disease. If this is confirmed and treatment is started before growth has stopped there may be a rapid growth spurt, enabling the child to catch up to normal size.

In addition to the usual finding of an iron-deficiency type of anaemia which has failed to respond to treatment coeliac disease can often be suspected because the blood film shows changes which are associated with atrophy of the spleen — fragmentation of cells, inclusions in the red cells called Howell-Jolly bodies, and cells called target cells because of their appearance of a rim of haemoglobin round the edge of the cells with a dot of staining in the centre. The cause of the disappearance or shrinkage of the spleen is not known, but it gives rise to these blood changes which are sufficiently characteristic of coeliac disease as to be helpful in diagnosis.

Confirmation of the diagnosis of gluten enteropathy requires the removal of tiny piece of the lining of the gut which is taken through a narrow tube passed into the upper part of the small intestine (jejunal biopsy).

Anaemia due to iron-deficiency

Age does not exclude the diagnosis. One of my patients was over 70 when I first saw her. She had a history of chronic iron-deficiency anaemia dating back many years, which had failed to respond to treatment. A careful examination of the blood film suggested a diagnosis of coeliac disease and jejunal biopsy confirmed this. She showed an excellent response to a gluten-free diet.

Treatment of iron deficiency

The most important aspect of treatment is to deal with any underlying cause, since in most cases treating the iron deficiency is merely treating a symptom.

There are many different preparations of iron which can be used. Unfortunately they all tend to have the same troublesome side-effects in some people, diarrhoea or constipation being the most important. Such symptoms, however, often disappear after a few days or can be overcome by reducing the daily dose. There is little evidence that the expensive 'slow-release' preparations have any advantages, and indeed some are much less effective than the simple cheap non-proprietary preparations ferrous sulphate, ferrous gluconate or ferrous fumarate. Preparations containing vitamin C are better absorbed but tend to have increased side-effects. None of the other additives in the way of minerals or vitamins has any additional benefit; they only add to the expense.

Symptoms improve rapidly with effective iron treatment, and changes in the tongue and nails are reversed. Difficulty in swallowing often improves symptomatically although the X-ray changes may persist.

Treatment needs to be continued for several months after the blood count has returned to normal in order to replenish iron stores, and if the underlying cause cannot be remedied (for example, in woman, with continued heavy menstrual loss) iron therapy may need to be prolonged indefinitely.

Coeliac disease needs to be treated with a strict gluten-free diet, which allows regeneration of the cells lining the jejunum and iron absorption will return to normal.

For the rare cases of real intolerance to iron, or severe malabsorption with poor cooperation in keeping to a gluten-free diet, iron may have to be given by injection, either by a course of injections into a muscle or into a vein. Although infrequent, serious reactions can occur with such injections which need to be given with great care, and only when there is a real indication.

Many oral iron preparations have a superficial resemblance to sweets, and great care should be taken to keep them out of reach since they are one of the commonest causes of accidental poisoning in children. Overdoses of iron are *extremely toxic*, producing vomiting, diarrhoea and collapse, and the condition requires *immediate* medical attention.

Prevention of iron deficiency

In recent years there has been much debate as to whether food should be fortified with iron in order to reduce the incidence of iron deficiency. There are however, many problems with iron fortification. First, the added iron may not be in an easily assimilable form; second, the iron may discolour some foods, change their taste or reduce their shelf life. Cereals have usually been chosen as the vehicle for added iron since they are widely consumed, but iron fortification adds to the cost of production, and in many parts of the world where iron deficiency is common cereals are not processed centrally. Furthermore, iron is poorly absorbed from cereals which have a high phytate content. Nevertheless, in Britain white flour has for several years been fortified to bring the iron content back to that of 85 per cent extraction; and a glance at the cereal packets on supermarket shelves shows that many manufacturers have taken it upon themselves to add iron to their products, usually at a level of 6.7 mg per 100 g of cereal.

The effectiveness of iron fortification programmes has yet

to be proved. An increased consumption of vitamin C-rich foods would probably be far more effective, particularly since in many countries where iron deficiency is common the dietary intake of iron is already very high though in unavailable form. Better health care and education, particularly directed at those most at risk, also has an important role in reducing iron deficiency.

There is one major objection to iron fortification programmes — the potential increased danger to those individuals who suffer from conditions associated with toxic iron overload.

Iron overload

The control of iron absorption according to the body needs is so efficient that it is difficult to produce toxic iron overload in a normal individual. It requires some additional factors to overcome the normal control of absorption.

Assessments of the normal amount of iron in storage differ for different populations, but it is generally accepted that there should be about 1000–1500 mg in reserve. This is present largely in the form of a soluble compound, ferritin, which is widely distributed throughout the body. When larger amounts of iron than can be stored as ferritin are present, aggregates of an insoluble compound, haemosiderin, are found in the tissues. Many grams of excess iron can be stored before damage to organs becomes clinically evident, but eventually if the accumulation of iron continues the result may be liver damage, diabetes and heart failure.

There are various causes of chronic iron overload. One is a genetically determined condition, haemochromatosis, in which the normal control of absorption of iron is impaired, and too much iron is absorbed. The defect, the nature of which is unknown, may increase absorption only two to three times the normal rate, but gradually over the years this leads to the accumulation of many grams of iron. The condition is

33

more common in men than in women, and symptoms seldom become evident till well on in adult life. In women onset of symptoms is delayed because of the protective effect of iron loss in menstruation. The effect of excess iron is widespread: most patients develop diabetes and liver damage, atrophy of the testes is also a feature, and a characteristic type of arthropathy (disorder of the joints) may occur.

This type of iron overload can be treated by removal of blood at frequent and regular intervals until the iron stores are depleted. Blood letting is then regulated according to measurements of the iron in the serum. If a person is diagnosed as suffering from haemochromatosis it is usual to examine other members of the family for evidence of the disorder so that any affected members may be treated before damage to the organs has occurred.

Apart from this genetic abnormality, excessive absorption of iron from the diet has long been a recognized problem among the Bantu of South Africa. Here it is attributed to the consumption of large amounts of beer fermented and stored in traditional iron pots. The acidity of the beer dissolves the iron from the pots, and both the acid and the alcohol keep the iron in a readily assimilable form. Many Bantu males may consume enough of this beer to give an intake of 50–100 mg of iron per day. Abandonment of the traditional pots, and changes in drinking habits from the illicit home brews to commercial beer, may be causing a reduction in the problem.

The high iron content of some local wines in northern Italy has been known to produce a similar problem of iron overload. Some village red wines in these regions have been found to have an iron content as high as 100 mg per litre though the average is more like 30 mg per litre.

Apart from iron accumulated by excessive iron absorption, overload may also occur as the result of multiple transfusions such as may be required in treatment of the chronic anaemias which do not respond to other treatment. Symptoms may develop after about 100 units of blood, the equivalent of some

Anaemia due to iron-deficiency

20 g of iron. In this situation removal of blood obviously cannot be used to treat the condition, but some improvement can be achieved by the use of iron chelating agents. These are substances which when given by injection can take up iron and increase its excretion, their use will be discussed further in relation to the blood condition thalassaemia (Chapter 8).

6

Anaemia due to lack of building materials: (2) vitamin B_{12} and folate deficiency

In order that the red cell may develop normally, in addition to the iron which is needed for manufacture of haemoglobin, two vitamins are essential, vitamin B_{12} and folic acid. Without one or other of these vitamins the nucleus of the primitive red cell cannot mature and bizarre abnormal cells called megaloblasts are found in the bone marrow. These cells are the essential characteristic of the group of anaemias described in this chapter, the megaloblastic anaemias. They include a number of conditions of which pernicious anaemia is probably the most well known.

The story of vitamin B_{12}

Cases of severe fatal anaemia, distinct from leukaemia, had been recognized since the middle of the last century. Addison, a Guy's hospital physician, is credited with the first description in 1855 of the anaemia now known as pernicious anaemia, although this term was not used until after the description in 1872 of fifteen cases of 'progressive perniciöser Anämie' by Biermer, a Swiss physician. In fact most of Biermer's cases were in malnourished young women and were associated with pregnancy, and were not the condition we now know as pernicious anaemia. The distinction was not made, however, until many years later.

In the latter part of the nineteenth century the German chemical industry discovered analine dyes, and their application to staining cells in specimens of tissue marked a big step

Anaemia due to vitamin and folate deficiency

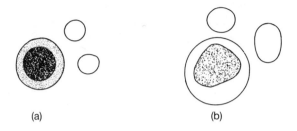

Fig. 7. (a) Normal developing red cell (erythroblast). (b) Abnormal developing red cell (megaloblast) in vitamin B_{12} or folate deficiency. It has an abnormal nucleus with a loose net-like appearance and has developed haemoglobin in the cytoplasm at a stage when the normal cell has none.

forward. Paul Ehrlich, who received the Nobel prize for both medicine and physiology, was an outstanding scientist of that time. Among his many contributions was the development of a stain which could be used on thin blood films to differentiate various cell types. In 1880, he reported that in some severe anaemias a large and unusual type of nucleated red cell occurred, to which he gave the term megaloblast (Fig. 7). The Ehrlich megaloblast became the essential diagnostic feature for distinguishing this group from other severe anaemias. But although the diagnosis was more precise, treatment remained ineffective.

In the 1920s, George Whipple the professor of pathology in Rochester, New York, was conducting a series of experiments investigating the regeneration of blood in dogs made anaemic by a carefully controlled programme of bleeding. He and his colleagues studied the effect of supplementing a basal diet of canned salmon and bread with a variety of animal and vege-table foods, and found that liver was the most effective in increasing haemoglobin production.

Although diet had been considered as possibly relevant in patients with pernicious anaemia, particularly as they sometimes had brief periods of temporary improvement, it remained for the Boston physician George Minot to consider this possibility more seriously. He himself suffered from diabetes and had become obsessional about details of diet. He took to making meticulous enquiries about the feeding habits of his patients with pernicious anaemia and concluded that many had a very limited diet, and in particular showed a distaste for meat. Bearing in mind Whipple's work he began, together with a colleague William Murphy, to study the effect of a diet rich in protein, including at least 120 g of meat and 120–240 g of liver daily. To take this must have required a considerable effort on the part of these frail, ill patients but the results were remarkable. All 45 of the first group of patients studied showed 'a prompt rapid and distinct remission of their anaemia coincident with at least rather marked symptomatic improvement'.

The response was regularly accompanied by a burst of young red cells (reticulocytes) appearing in the blood, reaching a peak in 4–10 days. In the subsequent search for the factor in liver which was involved in the response a reticulocytosis was used as a measure of the effectiveness of the different fractions. It was a laborious business as each new fraction had to be checked by the response in a patient with untreated pernicious anaemia since no animal model was available. British workers pursued this method right up to the time of the isolation of the pure substance by Lester Smith at Glaxo Laboratories in 1948. A few weeks earlier, guided by the finding that active fractions of liver also promoted growth of a microorganism (*Lactobacillus leichmannii*) American workers at the Merck Laboratories isolated the same factor which became known as vitamin B_{12}. The precise elucidation of its structure followed in 1956.

Minot's discovery in the year 1926, which transformed a previously fatal illness into a readily treatable one, stands out as the beginning of an era of scientific investigation of blood disorders as opposed to the hitherto largely descriptive era.

Anaemia due to vitamin and folate deficiency

Although pernicious anaemia could be controlled, the reason for the effectiveness of liver was not clear. It remained for another Boston physician, William Castle, to design a series of brilliantly simple experiments which demonstrated that the fundamental defect in pernicious anaemia was a lack of secretion of a factor in gastric juice which he called intrinsic factor (IF). The inspiration for Castle's work was derived from the knowledge that others had described a lack of secretion of gastric acid and pepsin (*Achylia gastrica*), associated with atrophy of the mucosal lining of the stomach in patients with pernicious anaemia. He was able to prove his theory of loss of secretion of an intrinsic factor by measuring the reticulocyte response in untreated patients with pernicious anaemia given normal gastric juice and beef muscle, either alone or in combination. Only in combination did they produce a response, and at the time Castle suggested that his intrinsic factor (IF) had to react with an extrinsic factor (EF) in meat to give a haemopoietic factor which would stimulate production of normal red cells and was stored in the liver. We now know that vitamin B_{12} fulfils the role of the extrinsic factor, and that the function of the intrinsic factor is to form a complex with B_{12} which resists digestion and passes through the intestine to the lower part of the small gut where the vitamin B_{12}–intrinsic factor complex becomes attached to the lining cells and the B_{12} is absorbed.

The fact that much of the progress outlined above was based on false assumptions does nothing to detract from the remarkable achievements over the years. We now know that Whipple's dogs responded because of the high content of iron in liver, and Minot's patients because of the 200–300 micrograms (μg) of vitamin B_{12} they were given daily, from which enough of the vitamin could be absorbed without the interaction with intrinsic factor. Some of the effect may also have been due to the folate content of the high liver diet (see below, p. 47).

Blood Disorders

Vitamin B_{12} is a remarkable substance. An injection of as little as 1 microgram (μg) (a millionth of a gram) can produce a response in a patient with untreated pernicious anaemia, and the total daily requirement is only 2–3 μg. The structure of the vitamin B_{12} molecule has some resemblance to the iron-containing molecule, haem. B_{12} also contains an atom of a metal, in this case cobalt. Some organisms require B_{12} for growth, others can make it if cobalt is available. This fact is made use of in the commercial production of vitamin B_{12} since the organism *Streptomyces griseus*, from which the antibiotic streptomycin is derived, also produces B_{12}. If radioactive cobalt is put into the culture medium of the streptomyces, vitamin B_{12} can be prepared with a radioactive label. Such material quickly advanced knowledge about the mechanism and site of absorption of vitamin B_{12}, as well as being useful in the diagnosis of B_{12} deficiency states and in methods for measuring intrinsic factor.

The discovery of folic acid

While chemists were attempting to refine and isolate the haemopoietic factor in liver another doctor, Lucy Wills, was working in India where megaloblastic anaemia was common, particularly in pregnancy. She discovered that the anaemia responded to treatment with a crude liver extract and to marmite (a yeast extract), but not to the relatively purified liver extracts active in the treatment of pernicious anaemia. The factor responsible was later found to be similar to one which promoted the growth of a bacillus (*Lactobacillus casei*), a discovery which formed the basis for the subsequent measurement of the level of the factor in blood and red cells. It was also similar to a substance isolated from yeast and from green plants, especially spinach, and which came to be known as folic acid. The naturally occurring forms (folates) in fact differ chemically from the substance folic acid, but the terms are often used as synonymous.

40

Anaemia due to vitamin and folate deficiency

At first when folic acid was isolated it was thought that it might be Castle's extrinsic factor (this was five years before the isolation of vitamin B_{12}), but it was soon evident that this was not so. It has, however, become clear that B_{12} and folates play an interrelated role in the normal development of nuclear material, and the absence of one or other is reflected in abnormalities of all rapidly dividing cells, the most characteristic changes being found in the bone marrow.

The discovery of the two vitamins and study of their metabolism has enabled a logical division and classification of the various causes of megaloblastic anaemia.

Vitamin B_{12} deficiency

Although the anaemia produced by lack of either vitamin B_{12} or folic acid is similar, the symptoms of the deficiencies differ in that B_{12} deficiency may in addition cause abnormalities in the nervous system. Often only the nerves outside the brain and spinal cord are affected, causing symptoms of tingling or numbness in the feet and a sensation of walking on cotton wool. More rarely the hands are also affected. In more severe cases some of the columns of nerves passing up the spinal cord to the brain may be damaged, resulting in an unsteady gait, loss of the sense of position, and the ability to detect vibration in a tuning fork held against the ankle or knee. This loss of sensation mainly affects the legs, but may extend up to involve the trunk and arms. The presence of such neurological abnormalities indicates a severe deficiency of vitamin B_{12} and was a common occurrence in the days before effective treatment.

Vitamin B_{12} deficiency may be caused by dietary deficiency, by malabsorption associated with lack of intrinsic factor or other conditions which interfere with absorption of B_{12}, or to the presence of organisms in the intestine which compete with the host for supplies of B_{12}.

Blood Disorders

Dietary deficiency of B_{12}

Vitamin B_{12} is found solely in foods of animal origin, the richest sources being liver, kidney and muscle. Several types of bacteria manufacture vitamin B_{12}, and ruminant animals, such as cattle and sheep, obtain their supplies of B_{12} from bacteria in the rumen, provided the metal cobalt (which is an essential part of the B_{12} molecule) is available in sufficient quantity. Bacteria in the large bowel, even in man, manufacture vitamin B_{12} and the habit of coprophagy (eating of faeces) in animals prevents them from developing B_{12} deficiency. Since man does not indulge in this habit, nor is he a ruminant, individuals who exist on a strict vegetarian diet (vegans) are prone to develop nutritional vitamin B_{12} deficiency. Vegetarian diets usually contain an abundance of folic acid, so the signs of B_{12} deficiency tend to be those affecting the nervous system rather than anaemia, the latter being prevented by folic acid. Less strict vegetarians who consume milk products and eggs are protected from vitamin B_{12} deficiency. Nutritional B_{12} deficiency is common in peoples who for religious reasons or because of poverty have a low intake, and it occurs frequently in Hindus, where it is often complicated by both folate and iron deficiency.

Reduced absorption of vitamin B_{12}

Pernicious anaemia is the classical prototype of vitamin B_{12} deficiency and is due to lack of intrinsic factor. The basic lesion of gastric atrophy, in which all the normal glands in the stomach lining have disappeared and the surface is smooth and the stomach wall thin, is at least in part genetically determined, but the type of inheritance is difficult to define since the anaemia seldom appears before the age of 40 (Fig. 8). A family history of pernicious anaemia is however found in about 20 per cent of cases. There may be a latent period, during which gastric atrophy and a diminishing secretion of intrinsic factor can be demonstrated for several years before

Anaemia due to vitamin and folate deficiency

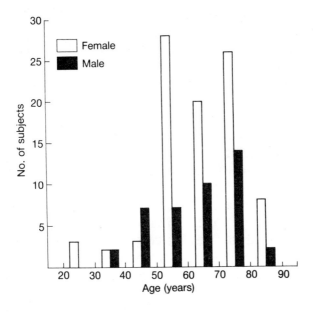

Fig. 8. Age and sex distribution of patients with pernicious anaemia in the Oxford region.

signs of vitamin B_{12} deficiency become apparent.

The incidence of pernicious anaemia is highest in northern European races, and areas to which they have emigrated, for example round the great lakes in America. In Britain the incidence is about one to two per 100 000 of the population. Fair hair and light eyes are common features as are premature greying of the hair and patchy loss of pigment in the skin (vitiligo). In most studies there is a female:male ratio of up to 2 to 1. Interestingly studies made some years ago on the distribution of pernicious anaemia in the United Kingdom showed the highest incidence in the previously depressed urban areas of the 1930s suggesting the possibility that iron deficiency, which was so common among women during the depression, might be a factor predisposing to the later development of

43

pernicious anaemia, and might also account for the higher female incidence.

In the early 1960s it became apparent that pernicious anaemia was one of a group of conditions associated with autoimmunity in which antibodies develop to the subject's own tissues — in the case of pernicious anaemia, to cells in the lining of the stomach and to intrinsic factor. Whether the antibodies are the cause of damage to the stomach leading to gastric atrophy, or are secondary to changes produced by some other factor, is still debatable. The tendency to form such autoantibodies seems to run in families.

In over 90 per cent of patients an antibody can be demonstrated in the serum to one of the cells in the upper part of the stomach, called the parietal cell, which normally produces both acid and intrinsic factor (gastric parietal cell or GPC antibody). In about 50 per cent antibody to intrinsic factor can also be found. Gastric parietal cell (GPC) antibodies are an indication of a damaged stomach lining but although they are most frequent in patients with pernicious anaemia, they are sometimes found in other conditions. The presence of intrinsic factor antibody, on the other hand is virtually diagnostic of pernicious anaemia.

Other autoimmune diseases occur with undue frequency in patients with pernicious anaemia and their families. This is particularly striking in the case of thyroid disease. In a study made in Oxford of 132 patients with pernicious anaemia 21 had a thyroid disorder. The thyroid may be overactive (thyrotoxicosis) or underactive (myxoedema), or it may be involved in an inflammatory autoimmune condition known as Hashimoto's disease. The thyroid trouble may antedate the anaemia or vice versa.

The clinical picture of pernicious anaemia is usually one of insidious onset, although an intercurrent infection sometimes produces a rapid worsening of the anaemia. A very frequent feature is soreness and burning of the tongue which may be smooth, red and show loss of the normal papillae. The pallor

Anaemia due to vitamin and folate deficiency

of anaemia is often accompanied by slight jaundice giving a characteristic 'lemon yellow' colour. Severe damage to nerves is seldom seen now as the diagnosis is usually made before the condition is far advanced, but there is often some numbness, or a 'pins and needles' sensation in the feet.

On the rare occasions when pernicious anaemia occurs in young people, there is often a complaint of sterility. This may respond dramatically to treatment of the vitamin B_{12} deficiency. One of my own patients conceived within a month of starting treatment after 17 barren years, another woman produced twins 9 months after recognition and treatment of her anaemia after 12 years of sterility. Male fertility may be similarly affected.

Some loss of appetite and weight often occur in the untreated patient, but indigestion requires careful investigation since cancer of the stomach is three to four times more common in pernicious anaemia than in the general population. It may occur before or after the diagnosis of pernicious anaemia, and this is one reason why patients should remain under regular supervision. The outlook on regular vitamin B_{12} treatment is otherwise excellent.

Since the upper part of the stomach is the sole area of production of intrinsic factor in the human, surgical removal of this part of the stomach inevitably results in a pernicious anaemia-like picture. However, since the daily requirement for vitamin B_{12} is only 2–3 μg, and the normal body stores amount to some 4000 μgs, it may take four or five years following the operation for signs of deficiency to become evident. Nevertheless, all patients who have had their whole stomach removed should be given vitamin B_{12} to prevent the later onset of anaemia.

If, during operation, the upper part of the stomach is preserved, megaloblastic anaemia follows in only about 6 per cent of cases. In such individuals the operation has usually been performed for a gastric ulcer, which is often associated with severe gastritic changes. Iron-deficiency anaemia is a far more frequent sequel to partial removal of the stomach than is megaloblastic anaemia, but in patients who develop a vitamin B_{12} deficiency the clinical picture is similar to that seen in true pernicious anaemia.

Since vitamin B_{12} is absorbed in the lower part of the small intestine, any disease of this area of bowel, or surgical removal for any reason, will reduce the capacity to absorb vitamin B_{12} and megaloblastic anaemia will be the result unless, as is common nowadays, vitamin B_{12} is given to prevent this occurring. One such condition is a chronic inflammatory disease of unknown cause called Crohn's disease. Although the Crohn's disease may itself cause reduced absorption of B_{12} malabsorption is more often due to removal of the affected part of the bowel. If more than about 17 cm of terminal small intestine is removed B_{12} absorption is significantly reduced.

Competition for vitamin B_{12}

An interesting group of megaloblastic anaemias is that in which bacteria compete for the supply of vitamin B_{12}, a situation that occurs in association with various anatomical abnormalities of the small gut. In older people weaknesses in the wall of the small intestine may allow sacs or pouches (diverticula) to develop. Blind loops of gut may be formed as a consequence of previous bypass operations, or strictures of the bowel may follow an episode of Crohn's disease. The normal small bowel harbours comparatively few bacteria, but stagnation of bowel contents in these abnormal conditions allows the proliferation of organisms which use up vitamin B_{12} and make it unavailable for absorption. Antibiotics which combat the bacteria may improve the B_{12} absorption temporarily but they cannot be continued indefinitely. Some cases are amenable to further surgical treatment, but most need to be treated as any other type of B_{12} deficiency with injections of the vitamin. These conditions are often complicated by iron deficiency.

Anaemia due to vitamin and folate deficiency

Another competitor for vitamin B_{12} is the fish tapeworm which is particularly common in Finland due to the partiality of the Finns for eating raw fish. The fish contain the larvae of this tapeworm in their muscles. The larva after ingestion by man develops and grows into an adult tapeworm, which may grow to as long as 3–10 metres. It has a remarkable capacity to take up vitamin B_{12} thus depriving its host of supplies of the vitamin. In a minority of patients this deprivation is sufficient to give rise to megaloblastic anaemia. Expulsion of the worm with anthelmintic drugs corrects the deficiency.

Folate deficiency

As already indicated, most of the early cases of severe anaemia described by Biermer (see above, p. 36) were not cases of pernicious anaemia, but can now be recognized as examples of folate deficiency.

Stores of folate in the body are far more limited than those of vitamin B_{12} and they can be exhausted in a matter of 3–4 months. The daily requirement is about 100–200 μgs, but this may be more than doubled in pregnancy. Most foods contain some folate, but the richest sources are liver, green vegetables, yeast, and nuts. A normal western diet provides something in the region of 400 μg per day but unlike vitamin B_{12}, folates are readily destroyed by cooking, especially at high temperatures, or with prolonged cooking. Cultural differences in the preparation of foods therefore have a considerable influence on the available folate.

Deficiency of folate tends to produce a more acute anaemia than that due to vitamin B_{12} deficiency. The white cells are often reduced to a level which causes symptoms such as ulcers in the mouth or on the tongue. The platelets may also be sufficiently reduced to give rise to purpura (a rash caused by bleeding into the skin from small capillaries). These two features are much rarer in vitamin B_{12} deficiency.

The most frequent cause of folate deficiency is malnutrition often associated with increased need, but malabsorption or interference with the action of folic acid can also cause a folate-related megaloblastic anaemia.

Dietary deficiency of folate

Diets lacking in folate are extremely common in some parts of the world such as India, and megaloblastic anaemia is very likely to occur especially in association with the increased needs of pregnancy. Megaloblastic anaemia of pregnancy is seldom seen in countries where folic acid is given as part of the routine antenatal care, but before the discovery of folic acid such anaemia developed quite frequently during the last three months of pregnancy or soon after childbirth, especially among the poorer sections of the community. The folate deficiency was often made worse by excessive vomiting, diarrhoea, intercurrent infection, toxaemia or twin pregnancy.

Others who are prone to nutritional deficiency of folate are elderly people living alone, who through poverty or lack of interest live on an inadequate diet, or chronic alcoholics and those suffering from diseases associated with loss of appetite.

Megaloblastic anaemia of infancy was recognized some years ago as a nutritional deficiency of folic acid, associated with the use of certain artificial milk foods. This type of megaloblastic anaemia is now reappearing with the fashion for substituting goat's milk for cow's milk in infants who appear to be allergic to the latter. Goat's milk is deficient in folate, and should not be given in these circumstances without appropriate supplementation.

Malabsorption of folate

Folates are absorbed from the upper part of the small intestine (duodenum and jejunum) therefore abnormalities of this area of the gut may interfere with absorption and lead to deficiency. Some gastrointestinal infections may lead to a condition known as 'post infective malabsorption'. This is particularly so with infection by a protozoan parasite called *Giardia lamblia*, which is a fairly frequent cause of traveller's diarrhoea. It is common in eastern Europe and is usually acquired through a contaminated water supply. Cysts of *Giardia* can be identified in the faeces in most cases, but some can only be diagnosed by passing a fine tube into the jejunum and sucking out some juice or by jejunal biopsy.

Tropical sprue is an allied condition and is now accepted as being a post-infective disorder. Before the days of antibiotic treatment and the discovery of folic acid, tropical sprue presented a very serious malabsorption picture and was fatal in a significant proportion of patients. The condition is seen mainly in people who live or have lived in an area where sprue is endemic — particularly India, the Far East and Middle East. Malabsorption of vitamin B_{12} as well as folate may occur as the bowel mucosal lining is extensively damaged. The symptoms respond well to the antibiotic tetracycline, combined with folic acid and vitamin B_{12}.

Coeliac disease (gluten enteropathy) has already been mentioned as a cause of iron deficiency (p.29). Because this condition causes changes in the upper small intestine it may also cause folate deficiency, which may be sufficiently severe to lead to megaloblastic anaemia. Sometimes, particularly in adolescent girls, the megaloblastic anaemia may be the predominant feature with little or no evidence of gastrointestinal symptoms. In others there is a more typical history of diarrhoea with bulky, offensive-smelling stools which are difficult to flush because of their high fat content.

Increased need for folate

Although megaloblastic anaemia of pregnancy is usually associated with malnutrition, the increased needs of pregnancy are equally important in causing folate deficiency. Any situation in which there is an increased turnover of red cells, as for example where the bone marrow is expanded to compensate for shortening of the lifespan of the cells, will also result in an increased requirement for folate. Folate deficiency is, therefore, quite often seen as a complication of other blood disorders.

Interference with the action of folate

The production of a folic acid deficiency and consequent megaloblastic anaemia occurs as an occasional complication of treatment with some drugs, notably some of those used in treatment of epilepsy. It is sometimes difficult to tell how far the anaemia is due to the drug or to associated nutritional deficiency, since many such epileptic subjects have severe and multiple fits and a poor diet. Treatment of the folate deficiency in addition to alleviating the anaemia usually results in reduction of the frequency of fits, and a general improvement in health, though in some cases an increased frequency of fits has been seen.

Folic acid antagonists are commonly used in the treatment of malignant blood disorders (see Chapter 12 on leukaemia) and will inevitably produce some megaloblastic change. This effect has to be carefully monitored, but is readily reversible.

The diagnosis of megaloblastic anaemia

As in the diagnosis of iron-deficiency anaemia, it is one thing to make a diagnosis of megaloblastic anaemia but quite another to determine which of the many causes may be responsible.

The characteristic blood picture is usually one in which there is great variation in size and shape of the red cells, but the majority are larger than normal and are well filled with haemoglobin (Plate 4a). In the megaloblastic anaemia of pregnancy, where the onset of anaemia may be very acute, such changes may not be so obvious and the true diagnosis can be overlooked.

The white cells and platelets may be reduced in number. In vitamin B_{12} deficiency this seldom produces symptoms, but in

Anaemia due to vitamin and folate deficiency

folic acid deficiency, especially that associated with coeliac disease, mouth and throat ulcers characteristic of a severe reduction in white cells (agranulocytosis) (plate 5) may occur and bruising or small haemorrhages (purpura) may be seen in the skin. The bone marrow in both vitamin B_{12} and folate deficiency is usually very cellular and shows the typical megaloblastic changes (Plate 4b).

Pernicious anaemia is the most likely cause of megaloblastic anaemia if a patient is over 40 years of age; this is particularly so if there is a family history of pernicious anaemia and/or thyroid disease, if there is early greying of the hair of the individual or in the family, or if the skin shows patchy areas of lack of pigment. Other causes of vitamin B_{12} deficiency can usually be ruled out from a careful history of the diet, and reference to any previous operations or abdominal conditions that might interfere with absorption.

Folate deficiency can occur at any age, but megaloblastic anaemia in younger people is more likely to be due to lack of folate than vitamin B_{12}. Again the dietary history, gastrointestinal symptoms, drug history or recent acute gastrointestinal infection may give a lead to the underlying diagnosis.

Vitamin B_{12} and folate can both be measured in the serum and, provided no treatment has been given, this will differentiate between the deficiencies although sometimes both levels are low. The serum can also be investigated for autoantibodies to the gastric parietal cell and intrinsic factor, the presence of which point to the diagnosis of pernicious anaemia.

The presence of acid in the gastric juice rules out pernicious anaemia, but a lack of acid can occur in other conditions. In addition to measuring the acid secretion, the secretion of intrinsic factor can be measured in gastric juice collected after an appropriate stimulus.

In investigating the cause of a vitamin B_{12} deficiency a test of absorption of radioactive B_{12} is often used. The absorption from a small dose of B_{12} given alone is compared with that from a dose given with intrinsic factor. Various diagnostic patterns are found. In dietary deficiency the absorption will be normal, since there is no defect in intrinsic factor secretion. In pernicious anaemia the absorption of B_{12} is grossly reduced but is improved with intrinsic factor. In abnormalities of the lower part of the intestine absorption of B_{12} is reduced and not improved by intrinsic factor. A similar situation is found in conditions where bacteria compete for the B_{12}, the so-called, 'blind loop' syndromes, but in these cases improvement in absorption may be produced by antibiotics.

Most patients who develop a megaloblastic anaemia will require radiological examinations of the stomach and/or bowel, and many will need to have the lining of the stomach or small bowel examined through an endoscope, a procedure in which a tube is passed, under light sedation, so that the interior of the organ can be seen, and if necessary a tiny portion of the lining removed (biopsy) for examination under the microscope. This is essential for the diagnosis of atrophy of the jejunum associated with gluten enteropathy, and may be helpful in some patients with post-infective malabsorption. It may also be used to confirm the gastric atrophy of pernicious anaemia, and to detect any malignant change in the stomach wall.

Treatment of megaloblastic anaemia

Vitamin B_{12} deficiency

Once it has been established that an anaemia is due to vitamin B_{12} deficiency treatment is started with injections of the vitamin. If anaemia is severe an injection is often given immediately after a blood sample has been taken. The results of further investigations will indicate whether this treatment is to be continued. Although the daily requirement is only 2–3 µg of vitamin B_{12} per day, and a response may be obtained with as little as 1 µg, it is usually to give large doses (1000 µg per week for a few weeks) in order to replenish fully the B_{12} stores as well as to bring about a remission in the anaemia. Treatment must be continued for the rest of the patient's life, although injections can be reduced in frequency to once a month or even once every 3 months. Vegans, who have normal secretion of intrinsic factor, can if they wish be treated by oral vitamin B_{12}, and this too should be continued so long as they remain strict vegetarians.

Some patients with pernicious anaemia wonder why they cannot be treated by an oral preparation of intrinsic factor. This was a method used at one time. Preparations of dried hog stomach containing intrinsic factor were given by mouth but some patients, after an initial good response, later failed to respond to treatment. It was the investigation of such patients which led to the discovery of intrinsic factor antibodies in patients with pernicious anaemia. Intrinsic factor has not been synthesized and no satisfactory therapeutic preparation is available.

Patients who refuse injections can be given very large doses of vitamin B_{12} by mouth (at least 100–250 μg daily) when enough may be absorbed without the combination with intrinsic factor. This is however, an expensive and unreliable method.

The response to treatment in a patient with B_{12} deficiency is quite remarkable. Within 6 hours the megaloblasts in the bone marrow are maturing normally, and there is an outpouring of reticulocytes which reach a peak in 6–7 days. Even before there is any noticeable change in the blood count there is a 'surge of wellbeing', and within 24 hours the appetite returns and the individual feels transformed — an incredible change from the gloomy outlook that existed before 1926.

As already indicated, patients with pernicious anaemia will remain well so long as they have regular treatment but they should be followed up because of the possibility of the development of a disorder of the thyroid gland, or the occasional complication of cancer of the stomach.

Blood Disorders

Folic acid deficiency

Treatment of folate deficiency is not usually a long-term requirement. Dietary deficiency may in many cases be remedied, and in megaloblastic anaemia of pregnancy treatment needs to be continued only until the blood has returned to normal. However, such anaemia tends to recur with subsequent pregnancies, and the patient should be given prophylactic folic acid during the second half of any further pregnancy. For treatment of anaemia the dose of folic acid is 5–15 μg daily, for prophylaxis in pregnancy 200–250 μg daily, usually given in combination with iron.

In megaloblastic anaemia associated with coeliac disease, folic acid will need to be continued indefinitely only if the patient is unwilling or unable to keep to a strict gluten-free diet. If this is possible the lining of the jejunum should regenerate, and folic acid absorption will return to normal.

Neither vitamin B_{12} nor folic acid will act as a 'general tonic', and there is no indication for treatment with either in the absence of a proven deficiency state. Folic acid should never be given to anyone who may also be deficient in vitamin B_{12}. This applies particularly to elderly people who, if they live alone, tend to pay little attention to their diet, and may develop folate deficiency; but they are also in the age group most likely to develop pernicious anaemia. Before folic acid is prescribed, the possibility of an underlying tendency to develop pernicious anaemia must be excluded, since folic acid can correct the anaemia but its use may lead to a rapid onset of damage to the nervous system if B_{12} deficiency is also present.

7

Anaemia due to shortened life of the red cells

In some blood disorders the life span of the red cells is seriously shortened. The early destruction of blood cells (haemolysis) may be caused in a variety of ways and the anaemias which result are grouped together as 'haemolytic anaemias'.

The earliest descriptions of such anaemias referred to the rarer types in which the red cells were destroyed while still in circulation (intravascular haemolysis), and the freed haemoglobin appeared in the urine. Towards the end of the last century, however, cases of anaemia with jaundice were recognized as also being due to increased red cell destruction. Later it was realized that some of these disorders were inherited and others were acquired.

A method introduced first in 1919 by Winifred Ashby who worked in the medical laboratories at the Mayo Clinic in America, was used in the early 1940s to investigate the life span of the red cells in various types of anaemia. The method was called differential agglutination (Fig. 9). Group O red cells

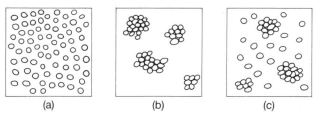

(a)   (b)   (c)

Fig. 9. The appearance of blood samples from a patient with group A red cells: (a) Normal appearance; (b) Sample treated with anti A; all the cells are clumped; (c) After transfusion with group O cells; sample treated with anti A — the patient's cells are clumped leaving the transfused cells free.

(universal donor cells) were transfused to anaemic patients of group A or B and in post transfusion blood samples the recipient cells were agglutinated (clumped together) by appropriate antisera leaving the unagglutinated donor group O cells free to be counted. Repeated blood samples in such experiments distinguished clearly between two types of haemolytic anaemia; one in which the transfused cells survived normally; the other in which they were rapidly destroyed. Furthermore, in the latter case the pattern indicated a random destruction of the transfused cells produced by some factor in the plasma of the patient acting on the cells. From such observations it was concluded that in some haemolytic anaemias the defect causing the haemolysis lay in the red cell itself, in other words an 'intrinsic defect' and in others in the red cell environment, that is an 'extrinsic defect', which affects both the patient's and normal transfused cells alike.

General features of haemolytic anaemias

Rapid blood destruction results in increased breakdown of haemoglobin with consequent increase in production of bile pigment. The liver may be unable to process the excess bile pigment, so the plasma becomes yellow and the patient jaundiced. In chronic haemolytic states the excess pigment may cause the formation of many small stones in the gall bladder (pigment stones).

In most haemolytic states the red cell breakdown occurs within the scavenging cells of the reticuloendothelial system but in some cases the red cells are destroyed while still in circulation (intravascular haemolysis). Free haemoglobin may then be found in the plasma (haemoglobinaemia) and in the urine (haemoglobinuria).

In an attempt to compensate for the shortened life of the red cells, production is increased by expansion of the red bone marrow, and in some severe congenital haemolytic anaemias this may be enough to cause bone deformities. Active marrow may even extend beyond the bones to form masses, for example, lining the chest cavity by extension from the ribs or alongside the backbone.

The development of anaemia depends on whether the increased production is sufficient to compensate for the shortened life of the red cells. If so, there may be little if any anaemia. With a healthy bone marrow production may be stepped up as much as eight times, and anaemia is unlikely unless the life span of the red cells is reduced to less than about two weeks.

Increased bone marrow activity is reflected in an increase in the proportion of reticulocytes released into the circulation (reticulocytosis) and nucleated red cells may sometimes be seen in the blood film.

With increased turnover of cells demands for folic acid are increased, and a folate deficiency may be added to the underlying disorder. Excessive destruction of cells may also lead to increased iron being deposited in the reticuloendothelial system.

In chronic haemolytic anaemias an enlarged spleen is usually a feature, and in some cases leg ulcers are a curious complication.

The congenital haemolytic anaemias

There are several conditions in which inherited abnormalities of the red cells make them less able to withstand the trauma of circulation. There may be defects in the cell membrane, lack of specific enzymes necessary to keep the cells intact or abnormalities in the structure of the haemoglobin within the cell.

Hereditary spherocytosis

Hereditary spherocytosis formerly known as acholuric jaundice, is the best-known example of haemolysis thought to be due to a red cell membrane defect, although exactly what

57

the abnormality is remains uncertain. As the name implies, instead of having the normal flexible biconcave disc shape the red cells are like tiny spheres which rupture very easily especially as they pass through the spleen (Plate 6).

The condition is inherited as a dominant character (see Chapter 3) although occasional apparently sporadic cases appear. The defect is present from birth, but is often not diagnosed till adult life, and some cases are so mild as to be discovered only during family studies. As the older name acholuric jaundice implies, jaundice is the most obvious feature and there may be little other disability. Anaemia tends not to be severe except at times of intercurrent infection when haemolysis may be increased. Certain viral infections particularly those due to human *parvovirus* may induce a temporary 'aplastic crisis' when red cell formation suddenly shuts down, and the continued haemolysis causes an acute anaemia. Such an infection may affect more than one member of a family and be responsible for 'familial crises'.

A history of recurrent mild jaundice dating from childhood together with a family history of the disease suggests the diagnosis. In addition to the characteristic spherocytic red cells which appear small and densely stained on the blood film, the reticulocytes are increased (except during an 'aplastic crisis'), and special tests will reveal the excessive fragility of the red cells.

It is important to recognize the underlying condition in patients who have gallstones, as if these are removed but the haemolytic state is left untreated further stones will form. Once the diagnosis has been established the spleen should be removed since the operation is virtually 100 per cent successful in relieving the anaemia and jaundice and prevents the formation of further gallstones. However, because removal of the spleen (splenectomy) increases the risk of infections, particularly in young children, the operation should in general be deferred at least until after 5 years of age (see below p. 151).

Anaemia due to shortened life of the red cells

Hereditary elliptocytosis

Hereditary elliptocytosis is another abnormality of the shape of red cells probably due to a membrane defect. In some people it causes no disability, but in others there is a variable degree of haemolytic anaemia. As the name implies the cells appear elliptical in shape in blood films. In patients with haemolysis, and if the spleen is enlarged, splenectomy may be beneficial.

Hereditary non-spherocytic haemolytic anaemias

Several hereditary haemolytic anaemias occur which do not have spherocytic cells in the blood and until relatively recently these were grouped together as 'hereditary non-spherocytic haemolytic anaemias' (HNSHA). In 1954 it was found that the spontaneous lysis (rupture of red cells and release of their contents), which normally occurs when a sample of blood is incubated overnight at body temperature, was in some cases of HNSHA not prevented by the addition of glucose, unlike blood from normal individuals or patients with hereditary spherocytosis. This led to investigations into the metabolism of red cells and the enzymes involved, and finally to the discovery of specific enzyme defects in some cases of HNSHA. There are several such defects but only two types are relatively common.

Pyruvate kinase deficiency   Deficiency of the enzyme pyruvate kinase is one. It is usually inherited as a recessive character (see Chapter 3) and is therefore only clinically obvious when inherited from both parents. The diagnosis depends on recognizing the general characteristics of a congenital haemolytic anaemia, and in establishing the particular biochemical abnormality in the red cells. Treatment consists mainly of transfusion when necessary, but when the disability is severe removal of the spleen is sometimes helpful.

Blood Disorders

Interestingly, an identical haemolytic anaemia is well recognized in Basenji dogs.

Glucose-6-phosphate-dehydrogenase (G6PD) deficiency The second type of relatively common enzyme deficiency is that of glucose-6-phosphate-dehydrogenase (G6PD). Sudden haemolytic episodes occurring after ingestion or even inhalation of the pollen of broad beans (*Vicia faba* or fava beans, hence the term favism) have been recognized since ancient times. The highest incidence of favism is in southern Italy, but the genetic distribution follows the progress of Alexander the Great even into northern India. The haemolytic episodes, which are characterized by their suddenness, severity and by haemoglobinuria, have been shown to be associated with an inherited lack of the red cell enzyme G6PD. In areas where the genetic defect is common, it has also been shown to be responsible for some cases of severe haemolysis in new born babies.

Another type of G6PD deficiency came to light first during the Second World War when some of the synthetic antimalarial drugs were found to cause sudden haemolytic episodes in some individuals. This was highlighted later in the Korean War when about 11 per cent of black American soldiers developed acute haemolysis and haemoglobinuria when given the antimalarial drug primaquine. The drug effect was shown to be due to an intrinsic defect of the red cells, which was later identified as G6PD deficiency. It is now realized that sensitivity is not confined to antimalarials, and a variety of drugs including sulphonamides and some analgesics can have the same effect.

Genetic mutations involving G6PD are common, particularly in the Mediterranean area and in people of black African origin. Many of the variants are silent, others cause clinical symptoms. The inheritance is sex-linked, the gene for the enzyme being carried on the X chromosome. In the presence of another normal X, as in heterozygous females, enough enzyme is usually produced to prevent anaemia, but males (XY) whose X chromosome carries the defective gene, or homozygous females in whom both X chromosomes are defective, are susceptible to haemolysis (see Chapter 3).

In G6PD deficiency treatment consists of avoiding as far as possible all drugs or other agents known to produce haemolysis. The attacks are self-limiting provided that the agent which produced the reaction is recognized, but an acute and severe haemolytic episode will require transfusion. Occasionally red cell destruction can cause kidney failure and treatment by dialysis may be needed.

The acquired haemolytic anaemias

The majority of haemolytic anaemias which appear first later in life and are not inherited are due to factors extrinsic to the red cells. Many are caused by coating of the red cells by an antibody which results in their rapid removal from circulation and destruction by reticuloendothelial cells. Others are caused by an immune reaction associated with a drug, or by direct chemical action on the red cells. Occasionally physical damage to the red cells may produce haemolysis.

Autoimmune haemolytic anaemia

The commonest type of acquired haemolytic anaemia is called autoimmune haemolytic anaemia (AHA) since, for reasons which are obscure, antibodies are developed against the patient's own red cells. Genetic susceptibility probably plays a part, since occasionally other members of the family show evidence of one of the other so-called autoimmune diseases such as thyroid disease or pernicious anaemia. In over half the cases of haemolytic anaemia there is no clear predisposing factor and the condition is described as 'idiopathic' (of no known cause). In the remainder the haemolysis is a symptom of other disease, particularly disorders of the lymphoid system such as chronic lymphatic leukaemia or Hodgkin's disease.

Blood Disorders

The anaemia may precede or follow the development of such a condition.

There are two well defined groups of AHA. In one the antibodies which are developed against the red cells are most active at body temperature (warm antibodies) and in the second the antibodies react most strongly in the cold (cold antibodies).

Warm antibody autoimmune haemolytic anaemia may occur at any age, but is commoner in older age groups and affects women more than men. In younger women it is likely to be part of the generalized autoimmune disease, systemic lupus erythematosus (SLE) (an inflammatory disease of connective tissue which affects many organs in the body).

The onset may be gradual or acute. The blood picture shows the general features of a haemolytic anaemia with a high reticulocyte count reflecting overactivity of the bone marrow. The patient is jaundiced, and the spleen is enlarged, though not usually to the degree found in long-standing congenital haemolytic anaemias unless there is some underlying disease involving the spleen. The diagnosis depends on the detection by special tests of antibody on the red cells or in the serum. The antibodies are often found to be directed at antigens of the Rh (rhesus) complex.

The course of warm antibody AHA is unpredictable. Treatment initially is with steroid drugs which suppress the immune response. Most patients show improvement with steroids, but the drug needs to be continued for at least 3–4 months after haemolysis has been arrested, although it may be possible to reduce the dosage or give treatment on alternate days to minimize the side-effects of fluid retention, gain in weight, 'mooning' of the face, and susceptibility to infection.

Some patients relapse when treatment is stopped, and if they can be maintained in remission only on undesirably large doses of steroids, removal of the spleen will have to be considered. The operation is not undertaken at first as the results are far less predictable then in congenital spherocytic anaemia (see p. 58).

Sometimes removal of the spleen results in recovery, in other cases it produces a partial response and allows control with smaller doses of steroids, but in a minority of patients it fails to give any benefit. In such cases immunosuppressive drugs such as cyclophosphamide or azathioprine are sometimes successful.

Those patients in whom the haemolytic anaemia is secondary to other disease are treated in the same way, but the final outcome is obviously influenced by that of the underlying disorder.

Haemolytic anaemia due to cold antibodies sometimes occurs as an acute episode associated with a chest infection caused by an organism called *Mycoplasma pneumoniae*. It is also seen occasionally with glandular fever. A weak antibody active at low temperatures against a person's own red cells is a normal finding, but these infections stimulate production of the antibody which both increases in strength and in thermal range so that it becomes active against the patient's own red cells even at room temperature. Symptoms of anaemia usually come on 10–15 days after the onset of the infection, and the blood recovers spontaneously, although occasionally the episode may be severe enough to require transfusion. Apart from this the patient needs to be kept warm until the rise in antibody subsides.

A chronic form of haemolytic anaemia associated with cold antibodies (chronic cold haemagglutinin disease or CHAD) is a disease of older people. The onset is usually gradual with episodes of jaundice, and sometimes haemoglobinuria occurring in cold weather. The person may complain of 'dead fingers' (Raynaud's phenomenon), and other exposed parts such as the ears and nose may become blue and cold. About a sixth of the cases are associated with a lymphoma (disorder of the lymphoid system) although the latter may not become apparent until some time after the diagnosis of the haemolytic anaemia.

The condition is often first suspected because of the difficulty in making a blood count and blood film. At room temperature the red cells run together in clumps (autoagglutination) and cannot be made to spread evenly. Precautions have to be taken to warm both the syringes into which blood is taken and the slides on which the blood films are made. The autoantibodies, although most active in the cold, are often still active at temperatures as high as 32 °C.

Episodes of haemolysis may be reduced by care in keeping warm at all times. If transfusion becomes necessary the blood must be warmed to body temperature and given slowly. Unlike warm antibody disease cold haemagglutinin disease is not improved by steroid treatment, but chlorambucil has possibly been useful in some cases.

Haemolytic disease of the newborn

A severe haemolytic anaemia occurring in newborn babies, or causing stillbirth, used to be a common condition with a high mortality. Its cause was unknown until the problem was solved in the early 1940s.

The discovery of the ABO blood groups made blood transfusions considerably safer, but they were still liable to be followed in some cases by unexplained reactions resulting in rapid destruction of the transfused cells. It was in the process of investigating such a reaction after a group O woman had been transfused with blood from her group O husband that two American workers, Levine and Stetson, observed in 1939 that the woman's serum clumped (agglutinated) her husband's red cells. A fact that was not appreciated at the time was that the woman had just delivered a stillborn baby who had haemolytic anaemia of the newborn. Levine subsequently put forward the theory that the baby might have inherited a red cell antigen from its father which the mother did not possess, and that she had produced an antibody which both caused the transfusion reaction and crossed the placenta causing the severe haemolytic anaemia in the child.

Subsequent investigations proved that this was true. Furthermore the antibody found by Levine was similar to that found by two other investigators, Landsteiner and Wiener, in rabbits and guinea-pigs immunized by rhesus monkey red cells. Human red cells which reacted with the antibody were therefore called rhesus-positive (Rh $_+$), and those not reacting rhesus-negative (Rh $_-$). The Rh groups have since been found to be part of a complex system, but the vast majority of cases of haemolytic disease of the newborn result from immunization by the commonest Rh factor (also called D).

Rh sensitization seldom affects a firstborn child unless the Rh-negative mother has been previously transfused with Rh-positive blood, but after one affected child there is a high probability of subsequent children also having the disease. The clinical picture takes various forms: anaemia, characterized by large numbers of nucleated red cells in the peripheral blood (hence the older name of erythroblastosis foetalis); anaemia plus jaundice which may be severe, and if the child survives leave residual symptoms of brain damage (kernicterus); or in the more severe cases a condition known as hydrops foetalis in which the placenta and newborn infant are grossly distended with fluid (oedematous). The most seriously affected cases result in stillbirth.

The discovery that this common conditions was due to an immune reaction in the mother opened the way to rational treatment and methods of prevention. It has become routine now to test all women as soon as possible after pregnancy has been confirmed for their ABO and Rh (D) groups. Any who have a history of transfusion, unexplained stillbirth or anaemia or jaundice in previous infants are tested for antibodies in their serum. These patients, and those who have been found to be Rh negative with an Rh-positive partner, are followed up, and their serum is tested at intervals to detect any appearance of, or rise in strength of, blood group antibody.

Blood Disorders

If such tests suggest that the child in the womb is affected, a sample of fluid from the amniotic sac is aspirated through the mother's abdomen (amniocentesis) in order to assess the severity of the haemolysis — indicated by the depth of yellow colour from bile pigment in the fluid. A decision may be taken to induce labour early when the indications are that a child is severely affected, but the dangers of prematurity make it unwise to do so before the 34th to 36th week of pregnancy.

At delivery a full assessment of the blood condition of the child is made on cord blood and a decision taken whether or not transfusion is necessary. This is usually an exchange transfusion — in other words, some of the baby's blood is withdrawn at the same time as normal blood is given. This method both removes antibody and damaged red cells from the baby and reduces the danger of overburdening the circulation. The blood condition needs to be watched carefully in the early days, as further exchange transfusions may be required especially if there are signs of increasing jaundice.

Since the cause of the anaemia is passage of antibody from the mother to the child through the placenta, anaemia does not recur if the child survives because the antibody gradually disappears.

People of blood group O have naturally occurring antiA and antiB antibodies in their serum. One might expect therefore, that a group O mother carrying a group A or B baby could produce a child with haemolytic disease. Although this may occur, the condition is usually very mild. ABO incompatibility in fact offers protection against Rh sensitization. This is thought to be due to rapid removal of fetal cells, which may leak across the placenta, by the naturally occurring antibody in the mother's blood. This concept has led to one of the most successful developments in preventive medicine.

The leakage of fetal cells, which causes immunization of the mother, is greatest at the time of delivery and separation of the placenta. Fetal cells may also get into the mother's circulation at the time of an abortion.

Anaemia due to shortened life of the red cells

If an Rh-negative woman who is at risk for immunization by an Rh-positive fetus is given an injection of antiRh (antiD) soon after an abortion or delivery, the fetal cells are removed rapidly and immunization is prevented in a very high proportion of cases. The dose of antiD to be given can be assessed by examination of a blood film from the mother. Special staining methods distinguish between her cells and those of the fetus, and the greater the number of fetal cells, the larger the dose of antiD required. Supplies of suitable antiD are obtained by immunization of Rh-negative volunteers.

This management has transformed a very common neonatal disease which previously occurred in some one in 180 pregnancies to less than a tenth of that number today.

Other acquired haemolytic anaemias

A great variety of drugs may occasionally produce a haemolytic anaemia, but the incidence of such reactions is rare compared with their widespread use. There are various ways in which red cells may be destroyed by drugs: some involve an abnormal immune response, others are the consequence of direct chemical action.

Immune drug-induced haemolytic anaemias

Three different varieties of this type of anaemia are recognized. With some drugs it is thought that the drug acts as an antigen inducing the formation of antibody. The antigen–antibody complex then becomes attached to the red cell membrane when a component of plasma called complement becomes bound to the complex and destroys the cell, so that haemolysis takes place while the cell is still in circulation (intravascular haemolysis). This type of reaction causes an acute episode which occurs usually with a second or subsequent course of the drug. The best-documented drug causing such a reaction is the antimony salt stibophen used for treating the parasitic disease, schistosomiasis (also known as bilharzia).

The second type of drug-induced haemolytic anaemia comes on more slowly, and usually only after a prolonged course of treatment at high dosage. Penicillin and related antibiotics may cause it by becoming bound to the red cell surface. This alone will not produce red cell destruction, but if an antibody to the drug has been induced this antibody will then react with the drug coating the red cell, with consequent damage to the cell.

A further type of reaction is seen in some patients taking the drug methyldopa for treatment of high blood pressure. The mechanism is not completely understood but the haemolytic anaemia is similar to autoimmune haemolytic anaemia. Antibodies against the red cells are found in some 15–20 per cent of patients taking methyldopa but haemolytic anaemia occurs in less than 1 per cent. As in autoimmune haemolytic anaemia the antibodies are often anti-Rh in type. The anaemia responds to treatment with corticosteroids which can be used if it is considered essential to continue treatment with methyldopa. However, as in all cases of drug-induced haemolytic anaemia it is preferable to withdraw the drug responsible as soon as possible, and replace it with a suitable alternative drug.

Chemical-induced haemolysis

An entirely different type of haemolysis is caused as a result of direct chemical action of some drugs on the red cell. The damage is caused by oxidation, either because of the strength of the oxidant action, or because the normal reducing power of the red cell which is dependent on enzymes is impaired, as in the hereditary enzyme defects already discussed (p. 60). Phenacetin and salazopyrin (the latter used in the treatment of colitis) are examples of drugs which have an oxidant action, but haemolysis is usually only evident after prolonged treatment. Other chemicals such as sodium chlorate, the weedkiller, which may be taken either accidentally or for self-poisoning, produce acute haemolysis and kidney failure.

The hallmarks of oxidant damage to the red cells are: first, the formation of a type of haemoglobin called methaemoglobin which is unable to fulfil the function of uptake and release of oxygen so the patient becomes cyanosed (blue); and second, the presence of inclusions called Heinz bodies in the red cells, which are aggregates of broken-down haemoglobin.

Haemolytic anaemia due to physical damage to red cells

Since the end of the last century the occasional occurrence of haemoglobinuria has been noted after running or walking in hard footware, a condition described as march haemoglobinuria (so called because the first case described developed in a soldier after a field march). The haemolysis has been shown to be due to mechanical trauma to the red cells in the blood-vessels of the feet. This emphasizes the need for properly designed running shoes with resilient soles if such haemolysis is to be avoided.

Since the development of cardiac surgery a new type of haemolytic anaemia has been recognized. Artificial heart valves often produce a minor degree of damage to red cells, but occasionally a severe haemolytic anaemia follows surgery. The haemolysis is intravascular and may produce haemoglobinuria. It is due to trauma from foreign material in a turbulent stream of blood, and if it continues the patient may need further surgery in an attempt to correct the situation.

Infections and haemolytic anaemia

Some infections result in the destruction of red cells, the most important being malaria. The type of malaria most likely to cause haemolytic anaemia is the malignant tertian variety caused by the parasite *Plasmodium falciparum*. The parasites are transmitted by the anopheles mosquito from host to host, but occasionally the malaria is acquired through transfusion of infected blood.

Blood Disorders

The parasites invade the red cells and develop there until they cause the cells to rupture. The degree of haemolysis is in part related to the number of parasitized cells but other factors may also be involved. Very severe and rapid haemolysis results in the picture of blackwater fever, the 'blackwater' being due to haemoglobin in the urine. Kidney failure and cerebral symptoms are common complications.

Because of the severity and seriousness of falciparum malaria it is extremely important that anyone visiting a malarial area should take regular and effective prophylactic treatment. Even a short stopover on a journey may be sufficient to acquire infection, and anyone who has recently travelled through a malarial area, if at all unwell, should be sure to report any possible exposure to mosquito bites so that appropriate examination of the blood may be made and treatment if indicated given as soon as possible. Unfortunately, increasing resistance to treatment acquired by malarial parasites is becoming a problem in some areas of the world.

In addition to malaria some bacterial infections may cause haemolysis, notably the organism responsible for gas gangrene (*Clostridium welchii*). The toxins produced by this organism have a direct haemolytic action on the red cells.

Paroxysmal nocturnal haemoglobinuria

Although this is a rare condition, it was one of the first types of haemolytic anaemia to be described. It has the striking and characteristic symptom of passing dark or reddish urine (haemoglobinuria) on rising from sleep, indicating intravascular haemolysis.

This is the only acquired haemolytic anaemia caused by an intrinsic defect in the red cells. Only a proportion of the red cells is defective suggesting that they have arisen from an abnormal group or clone of cells in the bone marrow, produced as a result of a change induced in one of the stem cells.

Paroxysmal nocturnal haemoglobinuria (PNH) is rare in

Anaemia due to shortened life of the red cells

childhood and affects mainly young adults, being slightly more common in women than men. In addition to recurrent attacks of haemoglobinuria the commonest symptom is attacks of abdominal pain, thought to be due to blocking of some of the smaller veins of the intestine. The major complications of the disorder are due to thromboses in larger vessels, particularly in the liver. The course is very variable often with long intervals between symptomatic attacks, which may be brought on by intercurrent infections.

Unlike other haemolytic anaemias, PNH is often associated with a hypo-rather than a hyperactive bone marrow, and the blood may show a reduced white count and platelets as well as anaemia. The reticulocyte count is seldom raised to the degree expected in a haemolytic anaemia. As a result of the haemoglobinuria there may be considerable loss of iron leading to a superimposed iron-deficiency anaemia. The diagnosis depends on special tests which show an increase in haemolysis of red cells in the presence of acidified serum.

Treatment is symptomatic, with transfusion when indicated by the level of the blood count. Because of the leakage of iron in the urine transfusions do not produce problems of iron overload. Transfusion reactions are common, but their incidence can be reduced by the use of red cells which have been separated from the plasma, white cells and platelets.

In a minority of cases the abnormal cells disappear and the condition recovers spontaneously. In a few cases the picture transforms to one of leukaemia. The majority, however, pursue a chronic course over a matter of years.

8

Inherited abnormalities of haemoglobin

Normal adult haemoglobin (HbA) consists of two paired chains of units (polypeptide chains) which are called alpha (α) and beta (β) chains. Before birth the fetus produces a different type of haemoglobin, fetal haemoglobin (HbF) in which the alpha chains are the same as in the adult, but two different chains, called gamma (γ) chains, are present in place of the beta chains. There is a gradual switch from gamma to beta chains after birth, but the changeover is not complete until about 3 months of age. In a few people, fetal haemoglobin (HbF) formation continues into adult life.

The discovery of the structure of haemoglobin, and analysis of the units which go to make up the molecule, have resulted in an explosion of knowledge about the causes of those anaemias which are the result of inherited defects of haemoglobin. There are two major groups: one in which one amino acid is substituted for another in one of the chains making up the molecule, (sickle cell anaemia being the most well-known example) and the other group, the thalassaemias, where there is a genetically determined imbalance in production of alpha and beta chains. In some parts of the world where both types of genetic defect are common there may be a combination of the two.

Figures obtained by the World Health Organization indicate that there may be 200–300 million carriers for the many varieties of disorder caused by haemoglobin abnormalities, and that every year 200 000–300 000 severely affected children are born. In some countries where infectious diseases have been brought under control these disorders have become a very important cause of ill-health.

Inherited abnormalities of haemoglobin

Sickle cell disease

In 1910 Dr Herrick, a Chicago physician, described a case of severe anaemia in a young black student from the West Indies and remarked on the 'peculiar elongated forms of the red corpuscles'. This was the first description of the now well-known condition, sickle cell anaemia.

Sickle cell anaemia is particularly important as it was the first instance in which an alteration in a single amino acid was found in one of the peptide chains of adult haemoglobin, thus introducing the concept of 'molecular disease'. Since this discovery hundreds of variants of haemoglobin have been described, some having little effect, others clinically disabling.

Studies on the distribution of sickle cell disease suggest that the abnormal gene may have originated as farback as neolithic times in Arabia, and spread by migrations to India and Africa, and by the slave trade to the West Indies and America. The incidence is particularly high in some areas of tropical Africa, where up to 20–25 per cent of the population are carriers of the sickle trait.

The minute change in the hemoglobin structure in sickle cell anaemia alters its behaviour profoundly. The sickle haemoglobin (HbS) transports oxygen normally but when it loses its oxygen, as in passage through capillaries and veins, the haemoglobin molecules align themselves in such a way that the red cells become stiff and sickle-shaped (Plate 7). For a time this 'sickling' is reversible as the cells are reoxygenated in arterial blood, but eventually the change becomes irreversible. In the process of sickling and unsickling the red cell membrane becomes damaged. In addition, the abnormally stiff cells do not pass easily through capillaries and veins and tend to cause obstruction to the blood flow. The symptoms of the disease are caused both by early destruction of the abnormal cells and blockage of blood-vessels.

People with sickle cell anaemia inherit the gene for the abnormal haemoglobin (HbS) from *both* parents, that is they are homozygous for HbS. Those who are heterozygous for HbS, in other words they inherit the abnormal gene from only one parent, have less than 50 per cent HbS, the remainder is normal adult haemoglobin. They are described as having sickle cell trait and show no clinical symptoms under normal circumstances. If, however, they are severely deprived of oxygen, for example by flying in unpressurized aircraft they may develop some mild temporary symptoms.

A patient with sickle cell anaemia (SS), on the other hand, suffers from a chronic haemolytic anaemia of varying degree. Crises of increased severity are common, precipitated particularly by infection or dehydration. The commonest type of crisis is a 'painful crisis' caused by blockage of small blood-vessels and characterized by severe pains in the limbs or back, often with areas of extreme tenderness over bones which may lead to an incorrect diagnosis of osteomyelitis (infection in the bone). The problem is made even more difficult by the fact that infection can occur at a site where blockage of vessels in the bones has led to areas of tissue death (infarct). Such areas of infarct may lead in later life to deformities, particularly in the hip and shoulder joints. Abdominal pain is sometimes a feature of painful crises and it may be severe enough to suggest an acute surgical emergency. It takes experience and courage on the part of the attending doctor to diagnose correctly and decide against an operation.

As in hereditary spherocytosis 'aplastic crises' may occur associated with viral infections, particularly human *parvovirus* infection. The blood count drops alarmingly and transfusion is needed urgently. Often more than one member of a family may be affected at the same time, and parents who have more than one child with sickle cell disease should be fully aware of this and be prepared to get immediate medical advice.

Another even more alarming type of crisis is the 'sequestration crisis'. Here a very large proportion of the red cells is trapped in the liver and spleen and these organs enlarge rapidly. This type of crisis occurs mainly in young children. Later in life the spleen usually atrophies due to repeated blockage of blood-vessels.

Apart from these problems, chronic leg ulcers are a feature in many cases, and painful swelling and distortion of fingers and toes may also occur.

In the absence of good medical care and readily available transfusion, few children with sickle cell anaemia survive beyond the first few years of life. This raises the question of how the gene can continue to remain so common rather than being gradually eliminated. The answer lies in a peculiar advantage of sickle cell haemoglobin. People with the sickle cell trait are more resistant to malaria than those with normal haemoglobin, and can survive better in areas where malaria is very common.

As already mentioned, people with less then 50 per cent of sickle cell haemoglobin (HbS) are not anaemic and have little or no disability when the remaining haemoglobin is normal adult haemoglobin (HbA). Young babies, even though they may be homozygous for sickle cell haemoglobin (SS) and have a high proportion of HbS, are temporarily protected from severe disease because of the persistence of fetal haemoglobin (HbF) in the early months of life. This modifying effect is seen also in some families who have an hereditary persistence of fetal haemoglobin (HbF) into adult life. On the other hand some other abnormal haemoglobins interact with sickle haemoglobin in such a way that even those with relatively low levels of HbS may show signs of severe disease. The sickling of cells which results from the alignment of the HbS and gelling of the molecules depends therefore on various factors: the percentage of HbS within the cells; the oxygenation of the cells; and the nature and amount of other haemoglobins within the cells.

From time to time various treatments have been suggested which might theoretically reduce the tendency for cells to sickle, but all have proved either ineffective or too toxic to be of use. Treatment therefore depends largely on recognizing the factors which cause crises, especially dehydration and infections. It has been suggested but not yet proved that since the type of parvovirus infection seen in cats and dogs can be effectively prevented by inoculation, similar preventive measures against human parvovirus might be applicable to children with sickle cell disease. Most adults have already acquired natural antibody to such infections.

Painful crises need to be treated with adequate pain killers. There is often a tendency to underestimate the severity of the pain, and sometimes some of the stronger drugs such as pethedine may be needed for a few days. The most important aspect of treatment is, however, to overcome dehydration which is almost always a feature. Plentiful fluid intake is essential, and if enough fluid cannot be taken by mouth it may need to be given by intravenous drip into a vein.

Transfusion to reduce the sickle cells to less than 40 per cent of the red cell population will prevent sickling, but it is not a practical long-term solution, and is better used as an emergency measure during a crisis, or to tide a patient over some particularly important limited period of time (as for example during a pregnancy).

The thalassaemias

The thalassaemias are among the commonest inherited blood diseases in the world. Over the centuries they must have accounted for the death of many millions of children, yet the clinical picture was not recognized as a specific disease until 1925, and then not in one of the areas of the world where the disorder is common but in the United States by a paediatrician, Thomas Cooley. Following his report more cases were found and the condition became known as Cooley's anaemia.

For some years it was thought that the anaemia was confined to people of Mediterranean extraction, and the name was changed to thalassaemia (from *thalassa*, the Greek for

Inherited abnormalities of haemoglobin

sea). It proved to be an inherited disorder, and the carrier or heterozygous state is recognizable as a very mild hypochromic anaemia (thalassaemia minor). Thalassaemia major is the severe homozygous form resulting from the marriage of two carriers of the abnormal gene. It is now known that thalassaemia occurs not only in people of Mediterranean extraction but also in the Middle East, the Indian subcontinent, Southeast Asia and Africa and among immigrant populations from these areas.

The thalassaemias are the result of defects in the genes controlling the manufacture of either alpha or beta-globin chains. If the gene for production of beta chains is abnormal, the resulting blood disorder is called beta-thalassaemia, and when the alpha chains are affected, it is known as alpha-thalassaemia. Reduced production of the affected globin chain leads to an excess of the other which tends to precipitate, particularly in the early nucleated red cells in the bone marrow. Beta-thalassaemia is the most common type in the Mediterranean area, and alpha-thalassaemia in South-east Asia, but both forms are present in many populations and interaction between the defective genes causes modification in the clinical picture.

The anaemia in thalassaemia is caused by several factors. The lack of normal haemoglobin production means that the mature red cells are deficient in haemoglobin (hypochromic). These cells also have a shortened life span so thalassaemia can be regarded as a haemolytic anaemia. However, a major factor in the anaemia is the very high proportion of the nucleated red cells in the bone marrow which never reach maturity, a condition called ineffective erythropoiesis. This results in an enormous proliferation of the bone marrow so that in severe thalassaemia, more than in any other condition, the bony cavities are expanded to accommodate the erythropoietic tissue causing distortion, particularly of the vault of the skull and facial bones. With the thinning of bones there is also a liability to fracture. The spleen becomes grossly enlarged which contributes to the anaemia both by a 'hyper-splenic' effect, and by the pooling of blood thus removing it from circulation. Finally, because of the enormously increased demand for folic acid, folate deficiency is a frequent complication which makes the anaemia worse.

The anaemia of thalassaemia major becomes apparent soon after birth. The child fails to thrive and is prone to infections. If the condition is untreated there is stunting of growth, and the developing bony distortion tends to give these children a similar mongoloid appearance (Plate 8). Their bellies become distended as the spleen and liver enlarge and they die young, usually of intercurrent infection.

This picture can be dramatically modified by regular and frequent transfusions, sufficient to suppress the abnormal bone marrow activity and to maintain the haemoglobin at near normal levels. Splenectomy usually becomes necessary in order to reduce the transfusion requirements but is deferred if possible until after the age of 5 years, and must be followed by treatment with prophylactic penicillin to reduce the likelihood of severe infections (see Chapter 17 on the spleen).

With access to good medical care, supervision at a centre familiar with the management of thalassaemia, and provision of adequate transfusion facilities, these children grow and mature reasonably normally, but tragically in their late teens or early 20s they develop fatal heart failure, liver disease or diabetes, all the result of toxic iron overload.

Each 500 ml of transfused blood adds some 200–250 mg of iron which cannot be excreted from the body when the trans-fused cells are ultimately destroyed. In well-transfused patients the iron overload is accounted for almost entirely by the transfused blood. In poorly transfused patients, however, a major factor is the continued ineffective erythropoiesis which, in some way which we do not yet fully understand, causes an excessive absorption of iron from food to a degree quite inappropriate to the high iron stores.

Some individuals with less severe forms of thalassaemia

Inherited abnormalities of haemoglobin

(thalassaemia intermedia) may be able to maintain a reasonable haemoglobin without transfusion except during worsening of the anaemia caused by infection. However, they too suffer from iron overload due to excess dietary iron absorption, although the toxic effects are usually not apparent until some years later than in patients with the major form of the anaemia.

Following the great improvement in outlook resulting from good transfusion regimes, great efforts have been made in recent years to reduce or prevent the iron overload. Iron is essential for the growth of many microorganisms and they are able to obtain it from their surroundings by secretion of special compounds which form soluble complexes with iron (sideramines). One such complex, desferrioxamine (DF) has been applied to the treatment of iron overload. This material has a remarkable affinity and specificity for iron, and is almost completely free from any toxicity. Unfortunately, it has to be given by injection, and the most effective method is by continuous infusion (through a needle inserted under the skin of the abdomen) for 8–12 hours, five to six times per week. The rate of injection is controlled by an automatic pump syringe. The infusion is usually set up at night to disrupt normal activity as little as possible. Clearly this is far from an ideal treatment requiring as it does intelligence and cooperation from both parents and children. The compliance of older children may be poor, teenagers in particular are understandably resentful of the limitations it places on their activities, and the prospect of needing treatment indefinitely is daunting. If, however, collaboration can be achieved, very significant amounts of iron are removed in the urine and faeces, the urine showing a rusty red colour from the excreted ferrioxamine.

The appropriate dose of desferrioxamine has to be assessed initially by measurements of the response to graded injections. Iron overload is often accompanied by vitamin C deficiency, and small doses of vitamin C (ascorbic acid) given regularly increase the effectiveness of the iron removal. It is important that the vitamin be given apart from meals so that it will not increase absorption of iron from food (see Chapter 5). Also, the daily amount should not exceed 100–200 mg, since very large doses have been thought to cause sudden heart failure in some patients with thalassaemia.

Current indications are that regular treatment with desferrioxamine is of benefit and should be started early in life. Several special centres are monitoring the long-term effects of treatment, and are constantly looking for better and more acceptable methods of management. As the child grows the dose of desferrioxamine will need to be adjusted, and progress must be assessed regularly by measuring the level of the iron complex ferritin in the blood, which reflects the level of the iron stores, and by tests of liver, heart, and pancreatic function.

It may be useful (though not as yet proven) to combine desferrioxamine treatment with a diet low in iron — in other words, vegetarian with a high proportion of foods from which iron is poorly absorbed, such as cereals and eggs, and to drink tea with all meals (see Chapter 5). It is important to avoid packaged foods such as breakfast cereals which have been supplemented with iron.

While the treatment outlined above may be acceptable in more affluent countries it is clearly unsuitable for many areas where thalassaemia is common. In countries like Cyprus, where the need for transfusion and desferrioxamine treatment is well recognized, the great expense involved uses up a major portion of the country's health budget.

Carriers of most forms of thalassaemia are easily diagnosed and several centres are now encouraging screening of populations at risk to detect carriers. Girls are urged to be tested before marriage or at first attendance at an antenatal clinic. If the tests are positive the partner is tested, and if he is also positive the chance of their child having a major form of thalassaemia is then raised together with the possibility of antenatal diagnosis. This can be made on a blood sample

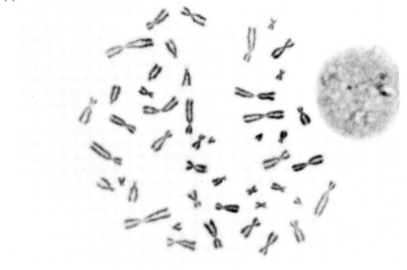

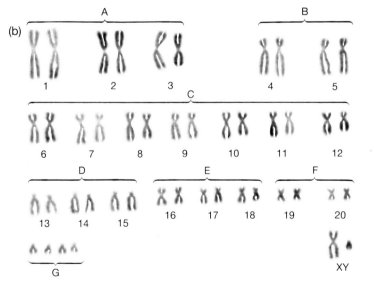

1. Chromosomes of a normal human male: (a) Special techniques are used to stimulate cell division and then to arrest the process; the cells are made to swell so that the chromosomes are separated and can be easily identified. (b) Chromosomes cut out from a photograph and arranged in numbered pairs. (Courtesy of Mr G. Breckon.)

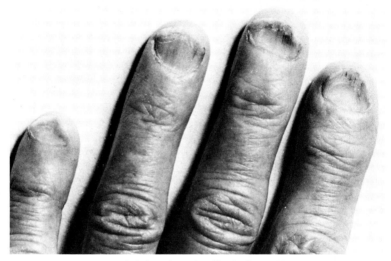

2. Spoon-shaped deformity of nails (koilonychia) in a woman with long-standing iron deficiency.

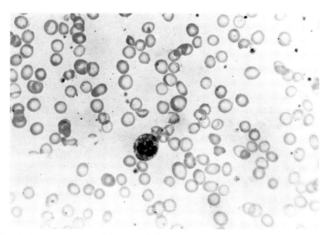

3. Blood from a case of iron-deficiency anaemia: the red cells are small and deficient in haemoglobin (microcytic hypochromic anaemia).

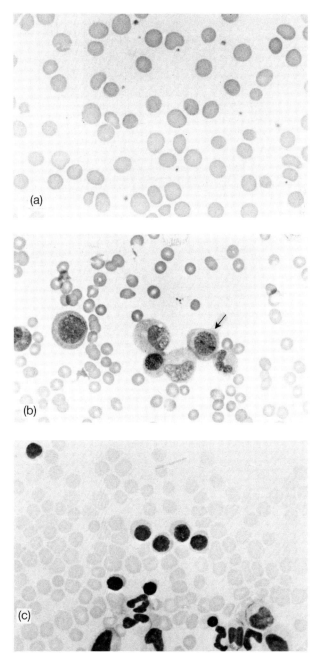

4. (a) Blood film from a patient with pernicious anaemia: the red cells are larger than normal and are well filled with haemoglobin (macrocytic hyperchromic). (b) Bone marrow from a patient with acute folate deficiency associated with pregnancy: the *arrow* indicates a typical megaloblast (large abnormal cell). (c) Response to treatment: the nucleated red cells are now much smaller and have a dense nucleus (normoblastic).

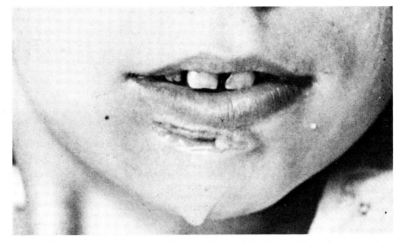

5. Severe penetrating mouth ulcer in a girl with coeliac disease and lack of white cells (agranulocytosis) due to folate deficiency. (Courtesy of Sir John Badenoch.)

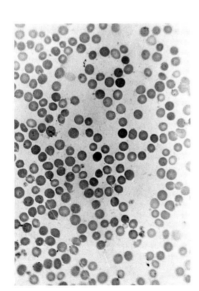

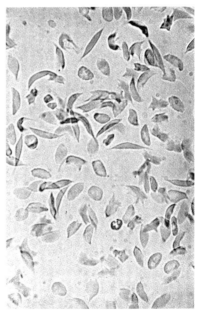

6. Blood film from a patient with hereditary spherocytosis: many red cells are small and appear densely stained because of their spherical shape.

7. Deoxygenated blood in sickle cell anaemia. (Courtesy of Professor E. Huehns and Blackwell Scientific Publications.)

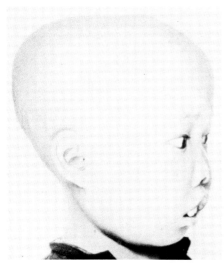

8. Deformity of the skull and face produced by expansion of the bone marrow in thalassaemia. (Courtesy of Professor D.J. Weatherall.)

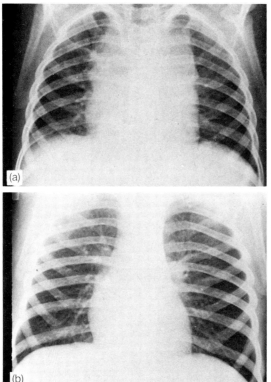

9. Chest X-rays of a 5-year-old boy with acute lymphoblastic leukaemia (ALL). The huge mass of glands disappeared rapidly on treatment with corticosteroids: (a) before, and (b) after treatment.

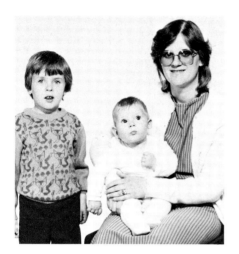

10. GC and her two children twelve years after the diagnosis of acute lymphoblastic leukaemia (ALL). (Courtesy of GC.)

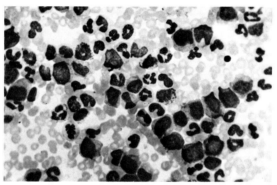

11. Blood film from a patient with chronic granulocytic leukaemia (CGL).

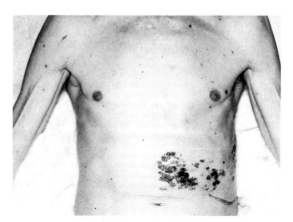

12. Haemorrhagic shingles in a patient with chronic lymphocytic leukaemia (CLL) and suppressed immunity; the rash has begun to spread and become generalized.

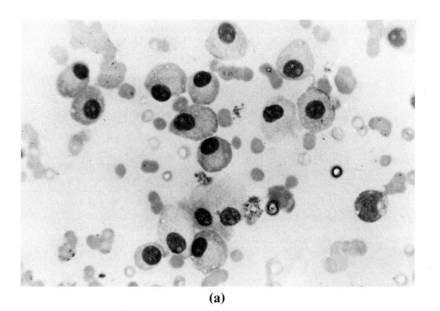

(a)

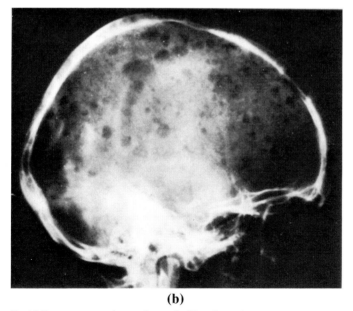

(b)

13. (a) Bone marrow in myeloma, infiltration with plasma cells which produce abnormal immunoglobulin. (b) Skull X-ray in myeloma showing areas of bone erosion.

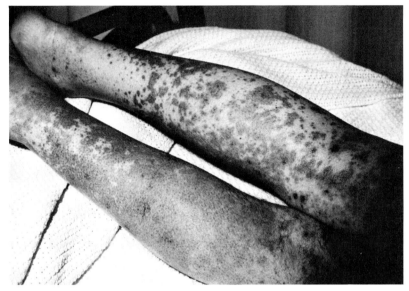

14. A patient with Henoch-Schönlein purpura showing a typical severe rash on the backs of the legs. (Courtesy of Dr C. Rizza.)

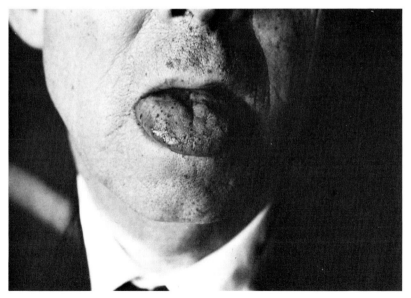

15. A man with hereditary haemorrhagic telangiectasia showing the characteristic lesions on the lips and the tongue. (Courtesy Dr C. Rizza.)

taken from the fetus from about the 18th week of pregnancy. The procedure in expert hands, carries a small risk of losing the baby, but the diagnosis is remarkably accurate and offers the parents reassurance that the child is normal or only a carrier of the trait, or the option of a therapeutic abortion if the prediction is one of serious disease.

Other techniques which are now being developed may well provide the possibility of diagnosis much earlier in pregnancy, which is clearly more acceptable if a therapeutic abortion is contemplated.

In countries where genetic counselling has been accepted by a high proportion of people at risk for producing a severely affected child, the incidence of the serious form of thalassaemia has fallen dramatically.

Similar genetic counselling and antenatal diagnosis is available for sickle cell disease, although this is not so widely practised since the natural history of sickle cell disease is much more variable.

9

Failure of blood formation

Aplastic anaemia

Aplastic anaemia is an uncommon condition in which there is failure of production of blood. All the blood cells are reduced (pancytopenia) and few if any early cells are found in the bone marrow.

In some cases the cause of the aplasia can be identified or at least suspected; in others no cause is found. Agents which are known to produce aplastic anaemia include radiation, benzene and related solvents, and several drugs. These include among others, drugs used in treating malignant disease whose aim is to damage cells, the antibiotic chloramphenicol, sulphonamides and allied chemicals, some anti-inflammatory drugs, gold salts, and some antimalarial drugs.

Radiation regularly produces some bone marrow damage but the extent of damage depends on the dose of radiation. The immediate effects are to destroy some cells and to damage the nuclear material of others. The shorter-lived cells, such as the white cells and platelets, are reduced soon after exposure, but because of the long life span of the red cells anaemia does not appear for several weeks. Provided the dose of radiation is limited recovery readily occurs and chronic aplasia is seldom seen as the result of acute exposure. It may, however, occur as a delayed effect after an interval of some years, and a proportion of such cases may go on later to develop leukaemia.

Benzene and related solvents are well recognized as agents which cause aplastic anaemia. Such solvents are widely used in industry, in dry-cleaning processes, and in the home and are particularly hazardous when employed in poorly ventilated conditions. Aplastic anaemia may be one of the dangers of

Failure of blood formation

glue-sniffing because of the deliberate inhalation of the solvent. As with irradiation there is usually a delay in onset of aplasia, which again may herald the development of leukaemia.

Most drugs which can cause aplastic anaemia affect the bone marrow seriously only in susceptible people. The damage may not occur with a first course of treatment, but on reintroduction at a later date. It is impossible to predict whether a patient will have an adverse reaction to any particular drug, but once having shown a reaction, it is extremely important that the same drug should not be used again. The fact that some drugs appear to need a 'sensitizing dose' suggests that some of the severe reactions may be immune in nature.

One of the problems in identifying a possible drug cause of aplasia is the fact that patients have often been taking, or have taken in the past, multiple drugs. The incidence of drug-induced aplasia is not high; for example, possibly of the order of one in 60 000 patients taking chloramphenicol, the drug most frequently recognized as associated with marrow damage, but drugs known to be potentially dangerous need to be prescribed with special care.

In recent years marrow aplasia has been recognized as a complication of some viral infections. Human *Parvovirus* has been especially implicated in the aplastic crises in the congenital haemolytic anaemias, but these do not go on to chronic aplasia. On the other hand, there are many reports of severe aplastic anaemia associated with hepatitis (virus liver disease). It probably has an incidence of one or two per 1000 cases of hepatitis and becomes apparent within 3 months of the onset of the infection. Such cases appear to have a particularly poor outlook.

Aplastic anaemia occurs at any age and in either sex. The symptoms depend on the degree to which the various blood cells are reduced. Bleeding due to lack of platelets is often the first symptom, with oozing from the gums, nose bleeds, prolonged menstrual bleeding and widespread bruising. The white cells are often less seriously reduced, but in severe aplastic anaemia they may reach dangerously low levels increasing the likelihood of complicating infections. Anaemia comes on more gradually as the marrow failure progresses and worn-out red cells are not replaced.

The clinical picture often suggests a diagnosis of leukaemia but the acellular bone marrow distinguishes the two conditions. If in doubt, a biopsy (a small core of bone marrow taken through a special wide needle) can be taken and sections prepared.

The diagnosis of aplastic anaemia is an ominous one. Figures vary for different series of patients but some 10–15 per cent may die within 3 months of diagnosis and over half within the first year. This poor outlook was one of the reasons for considering patients with aplastic anaemia for treatment by marrow transplantation, discussed below in Chapter 13.

If a suitable marrow donor cannot be found or there are no facilities for marrow transplant, treatment is aimed at supporting the patient with the hope of a spontaneous recovery. Bleeding is controlled by transfusion of platelets, but when repeated transfusions are required they may cease to become effective because platelet antibodies have been induced. In women it may be necessary to suppress menstruation by hormone treatment.

Control of infection is a major concern. If feasible, it is better to treat on an outpatient basis to reduce the possible contact with resistant organisms which are more common in hospital than at home. It is especially important to detect infections at an early stage and treat them appropriately. The danger arises particularly when the white count drops to a critical level below which infection is almost inevitable. The special care of such patients is discussed further in Chapter 12 on leukaemia.

Red cell transfusions are needed to raise the haemoglobin to reasonable levels, but with repeated transfusion the future hazard of iron overload has to be kept in mind since it is impossible for iron released from transfused cells to be excreted from the body.

The longer the patient survives the more likely is an eventual recovery, but complications from bleeding and infection take their toll.

There was hope at one time that treatment with anabolic steroids would improve marrow function. They may have a temporary effect, but toxicity and side-effects limit their use and there is little if any evidence of long-term improvement.

Recently, on the assumption that some aplastic anaemias may have an immune basis, the effect of immunosuppressive treatment has been tried using antilymphocytic globulin (ALG) which is aimed at destroying the lymphocytes responsible for the immune response. Some of the results with such treatment look promising.

Pure red cell aplasia

Although marrow failure usually affects all cell lines there are conditions in which one element only is affected. Pure red cell aplasia occurs as a rare congenital disorder which is diagnosed in infancy and goes by the name of the Diamond–Blackfan syndrome. The blood count is usually responsive to steroid treatment plus transfusions, but the necessity to maintain the treatment gives rise to many complications particularly retarded growth and susceptibility to infections. About a quarter of the children with this disorder eventually make a spontaneous recovery.

Acquired pure red cell aplasia is a different condition. In some cases a drug or a virus infection appears to be responsible. In others no cause is found. There is evidence that the condition is an autoimmune disease, and some patients respond to corticosteroids or immunosuppressive drugs. In about a third of the cases a tumour affecting the thymus (a gland situated behind the breastbone) is found. If such a tumour is present, surgical removal sometimes cures the anaemia.

Failure of production of white cells (agranulocytosis) and of platelets (thrombocytopenia) are discussed in Chapters 11 and 15.

10

Too much blood and related blood disorders

Polycythaemia

In normal healthy people the number of red cells is maintained at a stable level which is related to the oxygen demand of the tissues. Anything that reduces the supply of oxygen will stimulate production of the hormone, erythropoietin, which is responsible for control of red cell production. The result will be an increase in red cells, which will help to carry more oxygen to the tissues.

There are various physiological situations in which such an increase in red cells (polycythaemia) is found. It is part of the normal acclimatization process to high altitudes where the oxygen in the atmosphere is reduced. Polycythaemia is also associated with some lung conditions which reduce the capacity to take up oxygen, and with certain congenital heart defects in which part of the circulation bypasses the lungs (blue babies). In heavy smokers carbon monoxide accumulates in the blood and reduces the amount of oxygen available to the tissues. The polycythaemia resulting from all these conditions is called secondary polycythaemia and if the stimulus can be removed, for example by returning from a high attitude to sea level or by stopping smoking, the blood returns to normal.

There are some conditions in which the production of the hormone erythropoietin is inappropriately increased, resulting in polycythaemia. Since the main site of production of erythropoietin is the kidney, it is not surprising that this type of polycythaemia is most frequently associated with abnormalities of the kidney, particularly kidney tumours. Over production of erythropoietin is, however, found in only a small percentage of such cases. A brief period of poly-cythaemia which occurs after kidney transplant operations is attributed to a temporary increase in erythropoietin.

Polycythaemia vera

In the condition called polycythaemia rubra vera blood cell production is no longer under the control of erythropoietin. This is one of a group of disorders collectively termed myelo-proliferative diseases.

Polycythaemia vera is a blood disorder of older people and it is very rare under the age of 40. Most cases are diagnosed between 50 and 60 years of age and both men and women are affected. The cause is unknown, but something causes a change in one of the earliest bone marrow cells. This goes on to develop into an abnormal clone of cells which gradually replaces the normal cells.

The symptoms of the disease are often insidious in onset with vague complaints of tiredness, headaches, dizziness and weight loss. The appearance is plethoric and the eyes blood-shot. Sometimes, however, the condition is brought to light by a sudden complication such as a stroke or thrombosis, the result of the thick viscous blood sludging up in blood-vessels. One fairly common feature is caused by blockage of the tiny blood-vessels supplying the tips of the toes, one or more of which may become blue and cold. If the underlying disorder is not recognized and treated this may go on to gangrene and cause loss of tissue.

Somewhat paradoxically, as well as a tendency to throm-bosis there is an increased risk of bruising and bleeding due to defects in platelet function, so some patients may develop extensive bleeding under the skin brought on by little or no known injury.

Intolerable skin itching is a very frequent symptom which is almost diagnostic of polycythaemia vera. This is particularly related to warm conditions, such as in bed at night or in a bath.

Too much blood and related blood disorders

I have known patients having to go to the length of never washing more than a small area at any one time and then only in tepid water. The symptom is called the 'hot bath sign', and it is often the most resistant to treatment.

Gout is sometimes a complication of polycythaemia vera and a typical attack of acute gout may be the first symptom.

In addition to a very high colour of the face, hands, and feet, the eyes often appear bloodshot. In most cases the spleen is enlarged; sometimes large enough to cause discomfort.

Examination of the blood shows an increase in red cells and packed cell volume (PCV), which may be as high as 70 per cent and makes the blood thick and viscous. The haemoglobin may not be proportionately increased and indeed some patients have signs of tissue iron deficiency such as spoon-shaped nails or a smooth tongue, because all available iron has been used in the abnormal production of red cells. The white cells are usually only moderately increased. The platelets on the other hand are often very numerous and may appear both abnormal on the blood film, and function abnormally.

When all the typical features are present the diagnosis of polycythaemia vera is simple, but in some patients there may be doubt, particularly when the only blood abnormality is a moderate increase in packed cell volume. There is a condition called 'stress polycythaemia' which occurs typically in tense, overweight, middle-aged men with raised blood pressure. In such people the packed cell volume is high, but actual measurement of the total red cell mass shows it to be normal. At the same time the plasma volume is reduced thus concentrating the red cells and giving an apparent polycythaemia. In doubtful cases measurements of the blood, plasma and red cell volumes are essential to distinguish true from stress polycythaemia.

In addition, clearly all possible causes of secondary polycythaemia have to be eliminated by the history and appropriate investigations. Radiological investigations of the kidney are usually included when polycythaemia is first diagnosed, in order to eliminate erythropoietin producing conditions such as a kidney tumour.

Without treatment polycythaemia vera is a hazardous condition. There is every likelihood of death occurring within a few years as a result of a thrombosis or haemorrhage. Although there is no cure for the disorder the outlook has been immensely improved by carefully supervised treatment. The aim is to reduce the red blood cells and platelets to normal values, and to suppress the overactive bone marrow. In mild cases, or in the rare younger patient, treatment may be confined to the removal of excess blood by repeated blood letting. However, this only helps to reduce the thickness of the blood and does nothing to stop rapid regeneration of red cells. It has the additional disadvantage of making the patient iron deficient, and giving iron to combat this often makes the blood count very difficult to control.

The most usual forms of treatment aimed at suppressing the bone marrow are either injections of radioactive phosphorus (^{32}P) or tablets of one of the nitrogen mustard-like drugs called busulphan. Radioactive phosphorus is usually preferred and is simpler to control. It is injected into a vein, and becomes localized in the bone marrow where it irradiates the overactive marrow cells. An effect is seen quite soon on the white cells and platelets which have a relatively short lifespan, but the red cells show little difference until about 3 months after the injection. It may therefore be necessary over the first few weeks of treatment to take off a few pints of blood by vene-section in order to reduce the immediate dangers of thrombosis. Up to a pint of blood can safely be removed two or three times per week to bring the packed cell volume to between 45 and 50 per cent. A gain in weight is an early hopeful sign that treatment is effective and the disorder is being brought under control.

The blood count and general physical condition must be reviewed at regular intervals. If the first dose of radioactive phosphorus has not been quite enough to bring the blood to near normal a second dose may be given about 3 months after the first. Control, thereafter can usually be maintained by further treatment at intervals of a year or 18 months, or even longer.

Many patients now survive in good health for 15 or even 20 years from diagnosis, but there is an eventual tendency for the spleen to become progressively enlarged and the bone marrow to be replaced by fibrous tissue. This condition is called myelo-fibrosis. Alternatively an atypical leukaemia-like picture develops which is usually very resistant to any treatment. There has been much argument as to whether this is a natural termination of polycythaemia vera, or is more likely to occur as a result of treatment with either chemotherapy or radio-active phosphorus, but the fact remains that patients receiving such treatment usually enjoy many years of active life whereas untreated they would very probably have died or been disabled from a stroke, thrombosis, or haemorrhage.

Essential thrombocythaemia

This is another of the myeloproliferative disorders, the chief feature in the blood being an enormous increase in the numbers of platelets to five to ten times their normal value. They are also functionally abnormal. Although many patients have no symptoms, others suffer from a tendency both to bleed easily, and to obstruction of small blood-vessels, parti-cularly those of the toes and sometimes also the fingers. Strokes or mental confusion may be caused by blockage of small blood vessels in the brain.

The condition has many features in common with polycy-thaemia vera, and like it may go on to develop into a myelo-fibrotic picture with increasing enlargement of the spleen and marrow failure.

If there are no symptoms treatment may be unnecessary, otherwise it is on the same lines as for polycythaemia vera (see

p. 90). Antiplatelet drugs such as aspirin are sometimes used although it is doubtful if they are of much help.

Myelofibrosis

This condition has already been mentioned as a common termination of polycythaemia vera and essential thrombocythaemia. In the majority of people diagnosed as suffering from myelofibrosis there is, however, no preceding blood disorder. It is most common in older age groups with a peak incidence between 50 and 70 years of age and it affects both men and women. The cause of the condition is unknown and it may be recognized from changes in the blood for several years before producing any troublesome symptoms.

The bone marrow gradually becomes replaced with fibrous tissue and the spleen enlarges, often to an enormous degree. It is infiltrated with primitive blood forming cells a condition described as 'extramedullary haemopoiesis', meaning blood formation outside the bone marrow. This type of erythropoiesis is largely ineffective and does not sustain a normal blood count.

Apart from general symptoms of tiredness, malaise and weight loss the disorder may be brought to notice by discomfort from the sheer size of the spleen, or sometimes by sudden severe pain over the spleen due to blockage of one of the splenic blood vessels (splenic infarct). An inflammatory reaction on the surface of the blocked off area results in pain made worse on breathing, similar to that produced by pleurisy. In myelofibroses, as in polycythaemia vera and thrombocythaemia, extensive bruising or bleeding may occur and gout may also be a feature.

To begin with there is usually only a mild anaemia, but the diagnosis can be suspected from the abnormal appearance of the blood film, in which many of the red cells tend to be oval or rod-shaped or look like teardrops. Nucleated red cells and the occasional primitive white cell may also be seen in the blood film. Such a picture is described as a 'leucoerythroblastic anaemia' and it is a feature of extramedullary haemopoiesis. It is also sometimes seen where the bone marrow is infiltrated with cancer cells.

As the spleen gets larger it retains a large volume of blood, removing it from the general circulation and making the anaemia more apparent than real. The spleen may also reach such a size that it causes difficulty in breathing and heart problems.

There is no specific treatment for myelofibrosis but many patients remain in reasonable health for years with the help of occasional transfusions when the red cells drop too low for comfort. In more symptomatic patients careful treatment with one or other of the drugs busulphan or hydroxyurea has sometimes proved helpful.

When the massive size of the spleen becomes a problem the question is sometimes raised as to whether its removal would be of use — in some carefully selected cases it has proved beneficial, but in many others it has been unhelpful and hazardous.

11

White cells and infections

Granulocytes

As already explained the granulocytes are largely concerned with defence against infection. The normal response in most bacterial infections is an increase in granulocyte count. In children this increase may be very pronounced, up to ten or more times the normal value. On the other hand in the presence of severe generalized septicaemia the normal response may be absent, which is a bad sign.

When for any reason granulocytes are reduced in number or functionally defective the risk of infection is increased. Depression of the granulocytes (neutropenia) often occurs as a symptom of other blood disorders, or as a response to treatment of malignant diseases with irradiation or cytotoxic drugs, but isolated neutropenia is also well known as an adverse reaction to other drugs.

A severe reduction of white cells, almost to the point of disappearance from the blood, is described as acute agranulocytosis. The onset of this condition is usually dramatic with fever, prostration, severe mouth and throat ulceration, and sometimes ulceration round the anus. In many of the earliest descriptions of the disease, the outcome was a fatal septicaemia. The analgesic drug amidopyrine was incriminated in such cases, and with this drug and related ones such as phenylbutazone, the mechanism is now thought to be an immune response. Several other drugs including other pain-killing drugs, antimalarials, sulphonamides, antibiotics, and tranquillizers may occasionally produce agranulocytosis, probably by a direct suppressive effect on the bone marrow rather than by an abnormal immune response. As with aplastic anaemia it is usually impossible to predict such an adverse reaction, in a patient who has never previously shown a sensitivity to a particular drug or group of drugs.

Urgent supportive and antibiotic treatment is needed to prevent overwhelming infection in acute agranulocytosis, but if the patient survives the immediate danger of spreading infection and septicaemia the bone marrow usually recovers completely.

Amidopyrine, because of its association with agranulocytosis, is very seldom prescribed in the United Kingdom, but is still used fairly freely in other countries. As in aplastic anaemia, once patients have suffered an adverse reaction to a particular drug they should be warned not to take it again. Unfortunately such warnings may unwittingly be ignored, as for example with an elderly woman who had survived one attack of agranulocytosis, but suffered a second attack when her well-meaning neighbour offered her 'one or two of my red tablets which are wonderful for rheumatism'. They were phenylbutazone tablets, the drug responsible for the first episode, and this time they produced a fatal reaction.

In addition to acute agranulocytosis there are some rare inherited disorders in which neutropenia is a feature. One of these is 'cyclical neutropenia' in which episodes occur at fairly regular intervals, usually with about three weeks between attacks. The drop in granulocyte count may be sufficient to cause symptoms of fever, mouth ulceration, or infective lesions of the skin, all of which improve as the white cells return to normal.

Another more common type of neutropenia is associated with enlargement of the spleen. The mechanism is not really understood but the condition is referred to as 'hypersplenism', and it is a feature of some, but by no means all, disorders in which the spleen is much enlarged. Removal of the spleen may result in a return of the white cells to normal values but is indicated only if the neutropenia is severe enough to cause symptoms.

Blood Disorders

The normal function of granulocytes depends on their ability to move, to ingest foreign material and to kill bacteria, all of which in turn depend on extremely complex systems within the cells. It is, therefore, not surprising that some conditions have been described in which one or other of the normal functions is disturbed resulting in an increased liability to infection. Many are rare inherited abnormalities, but the growing interest in details of granulocyte behaviour and the development of more sophisticated tests are beginning to show that a number of diseases such as diabetes, ulcerative colitis and rheumatoid arthritis, may also show disturbances in white cell function.

Lymphocytes

An increase in lymphocytes (lymphocytosis) is a feature of certain infections. In assessing the significance of this it has to be remembered that under about two years of age children normally have a higher proportion of lymphocytes among the white cells than have adults. The best known examples of lymphocytosis produced by infections are viral diseases, such as glandular fever and german measles, but in whooping cough, a bacterial infection, a helpful diagnostic feature is a marked increase in lymphocytes.

Glandular fever (infectious mononucleosis).

Glandular fever is caused by a common virus of the herpes group called the Epstein-Barr virus (EB virus). In developing countries the infection is usually acquired very early in life and passes unnoticed. With higher standards of living, better hygiene and less overcrowding the infection is often not acquired until teenage or early adult life. The majority of older people show evidence of antibodies to the virus indicating a previous infection though it may have passed unnoticed. The virus is not easily spread from one person to another, but it is present in saliva, so glandular fever is sometimes referred to as the 'kissing disease' indicating the intimate contact necessary to pass on infection. The incubation period is probably about a month to six weeks. There may be a few days of feeling generally unwell with fever, headache, and loss of appetite before the onset of the characteristic sore throat. The throat is red, sometimes ulcerated and may be covered with a membrane or whitish secretion. The glands in the neck are enlarged and may be tender. Glands elsewhere, such as in the armpits and groins, may also increase in size and the spleen is usually enlarged. There may be transient skin rashes, but if the sore throat has been mistakenly diagnosed as a streptococcal infection, and the patient has been given ampicillin (an oral penicillin-like antibiotic) a widespread rash is induced in most cases. The liver is often involved in the infection, but jaundice is a feature in only about 10 per cent of patients.

The acute illness is usually over in about a week to ten days, but sometimes a period of depression and general lack of well-being follows before complete recovery.

The diagnosis is usually suspected from the clinical picture, but blood tests will confirm the suspicion. Many atypical lymphocytes are seen in the blood film. There is no anaemia, in the absence of the rare complication of an autoimmune haemolytic anaemia. The platelets may be reduced but not usually to a degree to cause symptoms. Further confirmation of the diagnosis depends on the results of special antibody tests.

Most cases require no special treatment except for relief of symptoms, for example, with simple drugs for headache and sore throat.

Cytomegalovirus infection

Another virus belonging to the herpes group causes an illness very similar to infectious mononucleosis with atypical lymphocytes in the blood; but it can be distinguished by isolation of the cytomegalovirus in the urine, or by finding a rising strength of antibody against the virus in the blood serum. A recognizable clinical illness is rare but most people have acquired the virus by adult life. Cytomegalovirus (CMV) infection has assumed far greater importance in recent years, because it may appear as a complication in patients who have their natural immunity suppressed by treatment, as in leukaemia or after bone marrow transplantation. A previous infection may become reactivated in such patients, or the infection may be introduced in one of the transfused blood products. This is difficult to avoid because of the wide distribution of the virus.

Disturbances of lymphocyte function

The lymphocytes are known to perform several functions concerned with immunity to infection. Defective function is a symptom of a number of blood disorders, notably the malignant disorders of lymph glands which are discussed later (Chapter 14). By far the commonest cause of suppression of immunity is, however, treatment with corticosteroids or cytotoxic drugs.

There are a number of rare inherited diseases characterised by functional disorders of the lymphocytes. These are known collectively as 'immune deficiency syndromes'. These congenital conditions are distinct from the 'acquired immune deficiency syndrome' (AIDS) which has received so much publicity recently. The indications are that AIDS is caused by infection with a virus allied to the human T-cell leukaemia virus. The infection affects mainly homosexuals, particularly those with several partners. In the few reported cases in women, their partners have generally also had homosexual contacts.

The AIDS virus can be transmitted by blood. Addicts are at special risk as they often inject drugs with shared syringes, which are not sterilised and may have been contaminated by infected blood. Patients receiving blood products, especially when these are prepared from large pools of plasma, are also at risk.

White cells and infections

Not everyone who acquires the virus will develop the severe loss of immunity which leads to death and which has produced so much public alarm, and the virus is extremely unlikely to be passed on by ordinary social contact.

Those at special risk for infection are urged not to become blood donors. Methods for detection of carriers of the virus and measures to make blood products safe are under active investigation.

12

The leukaemias

Popular fiction, films, and television have all played their part in familiarizing the public with leukaemia, often presenting a frightening image of the condition. All types of leukaemia are in fact quite rare but, since the decline of infectious diseases as the major causes of death in children in the developed countries, the malignant diseases, including leukaemia, have become the fourth most common cause of death in the under-15 age group.

Leukaemia is due to a change induced in one of the types of primitive blood cells. This leads to uncontrolled growth, the cells do not mature and normal marrow elements are gradually replaced by the abnormal cells which later invade the blood. This is why leukaemia is sometimes thought of as cancer of the blood.

Cases were first described in the middle of the last century. The name leukaemia was suggested by the creamy white appearance of the blood resulting from the combination of large numbers of white cells and anaemia. It gradually became clear that leukaemia was not a uniform disease but could be classified into various types; by the origin of the cells involved, for example lymphoid or myeloid, and into acute and chronic forms. The latter terms, though still used, are really outdated, since many patients with 'acute' leukaemia now have a better long-term outlook than some with the 'chronic' form of the disease.

Recently, with the use of more sophisticated and varied techniques more detailed classifications have been devised which are useful both for understanding more about the disease processes, and in designing the most appropriate treatment for a particular case.

The leukaemias

When someone develops leukaemia several questions come to mind. What causes it? Is it inherited? Is it infectious?

We do not yet know what leads to the development of leukaemia in a particular person, but we do know it is sometimes associated with certain factors, notably radiation injury, chemical damage, genetic factors, and viruses.

In the early days of X-ray diagnosis and treatment, when the hazards were unknown and little or no precaution was taken to screen the irradiation, the incidence of leukaemia was increased in radiologists, but this was reversed when adequate rules for protection were enforced.

Years ago the disabling condition of ankylosing spondylitis (a severe arthritis of the spine) was often treated with X-rays. This involved exposure of the bone marrow in the spine to irradiation. Many years later a follow-up study showed that leukaemia was nearly ten times more common in those treated by X-rays than in patients treated by other means.

The association of irradiation with leukaemia was brought to more general attention following the atomic bomb explosions in Japan in 1945. A rise in incidence of leukaemia was evident about three years later, reached a peak after five to six years, and then gradually declined. The incidence was related to the estimated dose of radiation, but it must be emphasized that of those people exposed to a harmful dose only about one in a thousand developed leukaemia, indicating a wide difference in individual susceptibility.

There is good evidence that leukaemia, like aplastic anaemia, can follow exposure to the solvent benzene. For example, in Istanbul, Turkey, in about 1961 shoemakers found that glue adhesives containing benzene were cheaper and more efficient than the glues they had used previously. Over 200 workers who appeared healthy but had been making shoes in unhygienic and poorly ventilated conditions were examined some years later. About a quarter of them showed some blood abnormality, and leukaemia was found to be at least twice as common as expected. As a result of these findings the use of benzene in shoemaking was prohibited.

Some of the drugs used in the treatment of malignant diseases may also induce leukaemia in some patients. Although this hazard is small compared with the beneficial effect of such drugs, it is constantly kept in mind when attempting to design more effective regimes of treatment.

Leukaemia is not inherited in the normal sense, but there are some inherited and congenital disorders which predispose towards the development of leukaemia. There is for example an increased incidence of leukaemia among children suffering from some of the rare congenital deficiencies of immunity. In Down's syndrome (mongolism), which is associated with a particular abnormality of one of the chromosomes, there is also a predisposition to leukaemia although this is less than was thought at one time. Twin studies have shown a slight increase in incidence of the second twin also developing the disease, but the unusually early age of onset suggests that some other factor induced the disorder in both twins before birth, rather than an hereditary influence.

In many animals, for example, mice, chicken, cattle, and cats, viruses have been identified as the cause of leukaemia. There is no evidence that these animal leukaemias can be transmitted to man, but there are indications that at least some types of human leukaemia may be caused by viruses. Recently a virus has been identified in a type of lymphoblastic leukaemia (the human T-cell leukaemia virus or HTLV). Such viruses may enter cells and become integrated into the genetic material leading to uncontrolled growth, or possibly they may remain latent for many years and are only activated by a trigger factor such as radiation. Whatever the part played by viruses, leukaemia cannot be considered as 'catching'. Although so-called 'clusters' of cases do occur, there is little as yet to suggest that these are associated with an infectious agent or that they could not have occurred by chance.

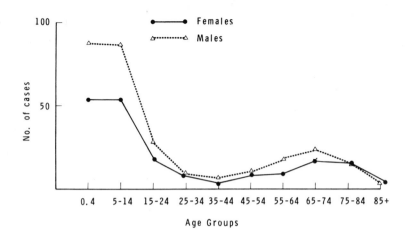

Fig. 10. Incidence of acute lymphoblastic leukaemia (ALL), expressed as new cases registered in England and Wales in 1973.

Acute leukaemia

Acute leukaemia has two peaks of incidence: in children below the age of 14; and in adults between 55 and 75 years. Childhood leukaemia is almost invariably a disorder of lymphoid cells (lymphoblastic leukaemia, or ALL) and is more common in boys than girls, whereas adult leukaemia in most cases involves one of the other types of primitive blood cells (acute non-lymphoblastic leukaemia, or ANLL) and affects both sexes equally. The incidence of new cases per year of ALL in the United Kingdom is about three per 100 000 in boys and two per 100 000 in girls; adult acute leukaemia occurs in between two to three per 100 000 (Figs. 10 and 11).

Most forms of acute leukaemia share the same symptoms, which are due to replacement of normal bone marrow by the leukaemic cells, and the consequent lack of normal white cells to deal with infection, and platelets to prevent bleeding.

Initial symptoms such as a sore throat and fever may be

103

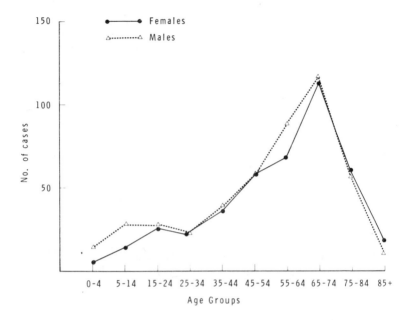

Fig. 11. Incidence of acute non-lymphoblastic leukaemia (ANLL) expressed as new cases registered in England and Wales in 1973.

mistaken for an ordinary infection, and only when the condition does not improve as expected, and other more serious symptoms develop such as extensive mouth ulcers, or widespread bruising and bleeding, is the suspicion of leukaemia aroused.

In lymphoblastic leukaemia, enlarged glands in the neck, armpits or groin may be obvious, and the spleen and liver may be enlarged. These features are much less common in ANLL. In one subtype of ALL (T-cell ALL) glands in the chest are often grossly enlarged. In the monocytic variety of ANLL two features are characteristic — a skin rash in the form of pinkish raised patches of leukaemic infiltration and marked swelling of the gums.

The diagnosis of leukaemia is usually clear from the blood

count. There is almost always anaemia and a low platelet count, but the white cell count can vary from very low to extremely high values. Even when the white cells are few in number a careful examination of the blood film will show some abnormal cells. The diagnosis is confirmed by examination of the bone marrow which shows masses of abnormal primitive cells ('blast' cells) replacing normal marrow.

Until 1948 a patient with acute leukaemia had no hope of recovery. The condition was rapidly progressive and death occurred within a few weeks or at most months. Then, because of some observations that folic acid might stimulate the growth of leukaemic cells, a group at Lederle Laboratories in the United States began to make a series of chemicals which were sufficiently like folic acid to be used by growing cells but were lethal to them (antimetabolites). One of these chemicals, aminopterin, was used by a group at Boston Childrens' Hospital in 16 cases of acute leukaemia. Ten showed 'evidences of improvement of important nature'. This was the breakthrough. With the development of new drugs, the outlook gradually improved so that 20 years on there were many reports of patients surviving for more than five years from the time of diagnosis, and it began to be possible to talk of 'curing' the disease.

Since any one physician will have under his care very few cases of leukaemia, special groups were set up, particularly in the United Kingdom, United States and France, where carefully controlled treatment on large numbers of patients could be assessed. These special centres have been the key to the advances in management, and the way forward has been possible only through the close cooperation of the patients and their families with such special teams.

Very few new drugs have been introduced since the early days of successful therapy, but modifications in the way they are used at different stages of the disease have sometimes produced surprisingly different results. The drugs used most commonly fall into various categories: corticosteroids, antimetabolites, plant extracts, products of fungal fermentation, enzymes and nitrogen mustard-like chemicals.

Corticosteroids When corticosteroids were first introduced they appeared to be so well tolerated that they were given for a wide variety of conditions, among them lymphomas and leukaemias. In acute lymphoblastic leukaemia dramatic improvement occurred in a high proportion of cases, and corticosteroids have remained of major importance in the treatment of this form of leukaemia (Plate 9).

Antimetabolites These are synthetic drugs designed to mimic one of the chemicals normally required for development of blood cells, but which are toxic to the cells. They include the folic acid antagonists, of which methotrexate (MTX) is the one now in general use, purine antagonists 6-mercaptopurine (6MP) and 6-thioguanine (6TG), and a pyrimidine analogue cytosine arabinoside (Ara C).

Plant extracts From the tropical periwinkle plant *Vinca rosea*, come the extracts vincristine (Oncovin) and vinblastine (Velbe) which stop cells dividing.

Fungal products The fermentation of a particular type of *Streptomyces* produces daunorubicin (Rubidomycin) and doxorubicin (Adriamycin) both of which are widely used, especially in ANLL.

Enzyme extract An enzyme, *L. asparaginase*, has been extracted from certain bacterial cultures. In interferes with the growth of leukaemia cells.

Nitrogen mustard-like chemicals (alkalating agents) During research in the Second World War blood changes produced by nitrogen mustard were noted. As a result many related compounds were developed which might be useful in treatment of malignant diseases, but less toxic than the original compound. These 'alkalating agents' have proved most useful in the treatment of the chronic leukaemias and lymphomas, but one, cyclophosphamide, is also sometimes used in acute leukaemia.

Some of the drugs (chemotherapeutic agents) are most useful in the earlier stages of treatment (induction of remission). Others are used for longer-term treatment. The aim of treatment is to eliminate all the abnormal cells and to allow regeneration of normal bone marrow. When all the signs of leukaemia have disappeared the patient is described as being 'in remission'. This does not, however, mean that all leukaemic cells have been destroyed, only that they can no longer be identified in the blood and bone marrow. For this reason further treatment is needed to try to get rid of the remaining cells and keep the condition under control. This is called 'consolidation and maintenance treatment'. Eventually a decision has to be made to stop all treatment with the hope that all will remain well.

Sometimes the leukaemia breaks through the maintenance treatment, or it may recur after stopping treatment (relapse). Attempts are then made to induce a second remission, which is often more difficult than at first.

Treatment of ALL

Remission is usually very easily brought about in acute lymphoblastic leukaemia, especially in children, by the use of corticosteroids and vincristine. Improvement is often noticed within a few days, and since these two drugs are not toxic to normal bone marrow, treatment may be continued at home, provided that there are no complications or infection. In almost all cases remission is complete by the end of 4 weeks.

It soon became apparent among the first patients to respond in this way that longer survival was often complicated by a form of meningitis due to leukaemic involvement of the nervous system. This led to the design of a second phase of treatment aimed at preventing the leukaemic meningitis (central nervous system, or CNS, prophylaxis). Few of the drugs used in treatment of leukaemia cross from the blood into the nervous system, which has been called a 'sanctuary site' since leukaemic cells survive there even when those in the bone marrow have been destroyed. CNS prophylaxis uses drugs such as methotrexate (MTX), which can be injected into the spinal fluid, and X-ray treatment to the head (cranial irradiation).

One of the unfortunate effects of both the vincristine given during induction treatment, and the cranial irradiation is that they cause temporary baldness. The hair will certainly grow again, but many youngsters find the baldness very disturbing and want to stay away from school and avoid company. Another feature which is seen in many children some 3–7 weeks after irradiation is the 'somnolence syndrome'. For a week or two the child is sleepy, lethargic, irritable and loses appetite, but this gradually passes off and leaves no after-effects.

After the completion of CNS prophylaxis the maintenance treatment is started. The drugs used are different from those used for the induction of remission and they need to be continued for $2\frac{1}{2}$–3 years. Some regimes include a brief course of 'reinduction' treatment at intervals during maintenance treatment.

If there are no signs of persistent disease treatment is stopped, but the patient is kept under continued careful supervision. After 4 years of continued first remission there is little likelihood of further trouble.

Girls on the whole have a better outlook than boys. This is partly due to the fact that some of the more resistant types of ALL are more common in boys, and also that the testes are another 'sanctuary site' in which leukaemic cells can persist. Of the commonest type of ALL in childhood about half can now be expected to be cured. Adult patients and some of the less common varieties of ALL have a rather less good outlook.

The leukaemias

Infections still account for serious complications during treatment. The drugs used during maintenance treatment lower immunity, particularly to viral infections — measles and chickenpox are especially dangerous. Any contact with either should be reported to the medical team immediately, so that an injection of immunoglobulin can be given to reduce the likelihood of developing infection. Measles unfortunately has no specific treatment. Chickenpox, and the related shingles on the other hand, can be treated with an antiviral drug, but this must be given early in the infection to be effective.

Treatment of ANLL

Acute non-lymphoblastic leukaemia (ANLL) does not respond to treatment so readily as ALL, and it has proved far more difficult to rid the blood and bone marrow of abnormal cells. Until very recently long-term survival was rare.

The rate of remission has improved since the adoption of much more drastic regimes but unfortunately these, while destroying the abnormal cells, also damage normal white cells and platelets so that the early weeks of treatment, before regeneration of normal bone marrow can occur, are fraught with the dangers of infection and bleeding. These very toxic regimes have been made possible only by the great improvements in supportive treatment in the form of measures to reduce the likelihood of infection (neutropenic regime), backed up by good bacteriological services and a wide range of antibiotics to treat infection, together with the availability of blood, platelets, and white cells for transfusion when indicated.

As has already been noted, when for any reason the granulocytes in the blood are severely reduced in number the chance of infection is greatly increased. In leukaemia, neutropenia is often part of the initial picture, but it is also the result of treatment.

The so-called neutropenic regime is designed to reduce the risks of a low white count. Everyone normally carries a huge number of bacteria on the skin and in the mouth, nose and bowel. When the white cells are reduced these organisms may become invaders. Thrush, a fungal infection, is another common problem in the mouth and throat. The routine consists of regular baths and use of an antiseptic in those areas particularly likely to harbour bacteria — armpits, groin, under the breasts, anal and vulval regions and between the toes. Mouthwashes are used every 2–4 hours followed by treatment against thrush.

Any damage to the mucous membranes or the skin may allow infection in, particularly in the anal area when an abrasion or crack may lead to ulceration. The motions need to be kept soft, and after the bowels are opened gentle washing with sterile cottonwool and an antiseptic should be used instead of toilet paper.

Some centres insist that these patients, while the granulocyte count remains below a critical level, should in addition be kept in strict isolation, given antibiotics to sterilize the bowel contents and eat only sterilized food. In patients undergoing bone marrow transplantation (see Chapter 13) this may be desirable, but in leukaemia it has only minimal advantages and increases psychological stress. The usual compromise is to nurse a neutropenic patient in a single room with emphasis on strict hygiene in the patient, staff, and visitors, and avoidance of foods such as fresh fruit and uncooked vegetables which normally carry many bacteria. Visitors or attendants with any kind of infection must, of course, be excluded.

Usually at least three drugs are used during the initial period of treatment of ANLL (induction treatment). They are given in courses of a few days at a time, with intervals of a week to 10 days or more between to allow some normal marrow recovery. The whole period of induction of remission usually lasts about 8 weeks, at the end of which the majority of patients will be in remission, particularly those in the younger age groups. CNS prophylaxis is not generally included in treatment although the need for it is under investigation.

The leukaemias

Some form of maintenance is usual for about a year after remission has been achieved. Although the outlook is gradually improving, only about 10 per cent of patients remain in remission for more than 3 years. Because of this relatively poor outlook ANLL is one of the conditions which is increasingly being treated by bone marrow transplantation following induction of first remission.

Psychological factors in treatment of leukaemia

While there have been remarkable advances, particularly in the treatment of ALL, so that some patients can now be considered cured, this is achieved at the cost of considerable and prolonged emotional strain for patients and their families. The treatment itself and the hazards involved, mean that special expertise in management is required, and this often means that patients must attend a centre which may be far from home.

The diagnosis, however sympathetically explained, comes as a shock, but most will agree that it cannot and should not be concealed when so much depends on keeping to strict treatment regimes, and on understanding the possible complications along the line. Even quite young children may need a simple explanation of why they need treatment.

The parents of a child with leukaemia should see the doctor together, so that they both know what the prospects are. In the initial emotional upheaval there is the possibility of great confusion if one parent only discusses the problem. It is often difficult at first to understand the issues fully, but staff should be available at any time to help. At many centres parents have formed associations which give support and help to others.

Difficulties often arise at home with other children who may develop behaviour disorders when one or both parents become too involved with the leukaemic child. There may be a great temptation to lavish special attention, to indulge the child, or to make unattainable promises. It takes much courage and control to avoid this and to strike the right balance.

Blood Disorders

It is often difficult to accept that children with leukaemia should be allowed to lead as normal a life as possible. There is no need to keep them away from school except when there are epidemics of illness (especially chickenpox or measles), but it is wise for the teachers to be taken into the confidence of parents so that they will understand the need for absences during visits to hospital. Depression and anxiety are common in leukaemic children especially if anxious parents curtail their activities unnecessarily.

Adults with leukaemia need to share their anxieties with close relatives and friends. If a marriage has been strained before the illness, breakdown of the relationship may follow. On the other hand, many couples have found some compensation in being brought closer together by the mutual problem.

Like children adults also need to resume all normal activity as soon as their condition allows. One of my most courageous patients was back playing football very shortly after a very stormy induction of remission. His positive attitude and determination were an example to others.

Those who get safely through all the hazards and can be considered cured have remarkably little in the way of after-effects. In children who have had cranial irradiation at an early age, there is occasionally some early learning difficulty, especially in mathematical skills, but there are now many examples of youngsters who have done well at school and university. Growth is usually normal and both sexes mature normally although fertility may be reduced, at least for some years. The seriousness of this problem can only be assessed when increasing numbers of leukaemic children reach maturity. Several formerly leukaemic girls have, however, now produced normal healthy children (Plate 10), and some boys have later fathered children.

Chronic granulocytic leukaemia (CGL)

This type of leukaemia is rarer than acute leukaemia. It occurs most commonly over the age of fifty (Fig. 12). At first there may be few symptoms and in many cases the diagnosis is made by chance. In others there are vague complaints of tiredness, weight loss, or abdominal discomfort related to enlargement of the spleen. Occasionally a sudden episode of severe abdominal pain, the result of blockage of a blood vessel in the spleen (splenic infarct), brings the condition to light. The most characteristic finding on examination is enlargement of the spleen, which is sometimes massive.

At the onset there is usually a moderate anaemia and a raised white count, often ten to 40 times the normal value or even higher. Very high platelet counts are common too. The blood film (Plate 11) shows a picture very different from that

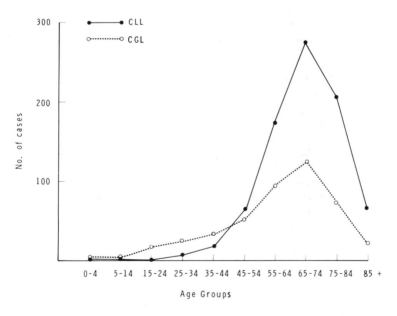

Fig. 12. Incidence of chronic granulocytic leukaemia (CGL) and chronic lymphocytic leukaemia (CLL) in different age groups, expressed as new cases registered in England and Wales in 1973.

of acute leukaemia. Most of the cells are fairly mature and have developed granules; many are fully mature. The primitive 'blast cells' which predominate in acute leukaemia are few in number. Although the cells have arisen from an abnormal clone they are still capable of killing bacteria, so infection is not a problem. Nearly all cases of CGL have a specific chromosome abnormality called the Ph_1 (Philadelphia) chromosome, which nearly always persists even when the condition is brought under control by treatment.

There are two phases to the illness. During the first phase treatment can relieve all symptoms, shrink the spleen and return the blood to normal values, so the patient feels fit and healthy again. Sooner or later, however, the disease picture changes to a more aggressive phase. This takes the form either of an acute type of leukaemia or more often a state where the spleen progressively enlarges, and wasting, weakness, fever and an anaemia which does not respond to treatment lead to death.

Treatment of the chronic phase is usually with busulphan (one of the nitrogen mustard-like agents). It is remarkably effective and well tolerated but the dosage needs to be carefully controlled by regular blood counts, since busulphan can damage the bone marrow and produce aplasia which may be slow to recover. Busulphan frequently produces a darkening of the skin which is harmless, very occasionally it produces fibrosis in the lungs which is serious.

Once the disease has become more aggressive little can be done beyond supportive care. Occasionally some of the drugs used in treatment of other forms of acute leukaemia produce a temporary remission in a 'blast crisis', but usually they are of little help.

The outlook from the time of diagnosis varies from months to 12 to 15 years or, exceptionally, to 20 years but the average is only about three years and only about 15 per cent of patients live for more than 5 years. Because of the inability to cure CGL with present treatment this condition is increasingly

being considered for treatment by bone marrow transplantation.

Chronic lymphatic leukaemia (CLL)

In contrast to other forms of leukaemia there are no clues as to
possible causes of chronic lymphatic leukaemia. The condition is more allied to some of the disorders of the lymph
glands than to any other form of leukaemia. It is more
common in men, and is a disease of later life being rare below
the age of 40 (Fig. 12).

In about a quarter of the patients the condition is
completely symptomless and is discovered only by chance. In
others there may be general symptoms of malaise, weight loss
or fever and enlarged lymph glands or lumps in the skin may
have been noticed. There may be a history of frequent chest
infections associated with a general increased susceptibility to
infection; the result of a failure in function of the abnormal
lymphocytes in this condition. Examination usually reveals
some enlargement of both lymph nodes and spleen, and occasionally infiltration of the skin.

The diagnosis is made on the blood which shows some
anaemia and an increased proportion of lymphoid cells. The
total white count is very variable, but a high proportion of
lymphocytes is always present. The bone marrow also shows
an increase in lymphoid cells.

Patients without symptoms are usually just kept under
observation and may never require any treatment. They may
survive for 20 years or more with no apparent progression
of the disease. Others develop troublesome enlargement of
glands or increasing anaemia. Localized large groups of
glands can be shrunk by radiotherapy, but more generalized
symptoms require treatment which usually consists of one of
the alkalating agents (chlorambucil) with or without the
addition of corticosteroids.

Some patients develop an autoimmune haemolytic anaemia

(see p. 63) or thrombocytopenia (see p. 141) which generally respond to corticosteroids, but may require splenectomy. Occasionally the spleen is so grossly enlarged that a large amount of blood is trapped in it (splenic pooling), or its sheer size may cause great discomfort. Removal in these circumstances may give great relief of symptoms.

Infections are always a hazard in CLL because of the reduced immunity. Viral and fungal infections are particularly dangerous. Shingles (herpes zoster) is a common complication and unless treated promptly may spread and become generalized (Plate 12). There are now antiviral agents which will help to arrest the spread and cut short the infection, so it is important that any suggestion of shingles should be reported to a doctor immediately.

The general outlook is extremely variable and often unpredictable. In some patients the condition appears static; in others it may be fairly rapidly progressive with increasing anaemia and a diminishing response to treatment.

13

Bone marrow transplantation

Bone marrow transplantation has over the past 15 years been used increasingly in various blood disorders. The feasibility of successful marrow transplant was first shown in animals but it was the discovery of the 'histocompatibility antigens' which made possible the application to man.

In 1952 some patients who had received multiple blood transfusions were shown to have developed antibodies to white cells. This was the beginning of the definition of the HLA (human leucocyte antigen) system which has become of fundamental importance in matching donors of transplants to recipients. The antigens are not only carried on white cells but also on most tissue cells (hence the term histocompatibility antigen hist meaning tissue), and they are inherited. There are a great many alternative genes at each of the sites making up the HLA·complex, and the chances of finding an unrelated donor of identical type are extremely remote. The genes are, however, closely linked on one chromosome and are inherited together as a haplotype (see Chapter 3). If the haplotypes of the mother are represented as ab and the father cd there can be only four possible combinations in the children, ac, bc, ad and bd, so among brothers and sisters there is a one in four chance of finding a donor of the same type. The ideal donor of course, is an identical twin.

In addition to having a suitably matched donor, success in bone marrow transplant depends on preparing the recipient with treatment designed to abolish all the cells which are responsible for causing an immune reaction to any foreign tissue, resulting in rejection of the graft. In malignant blood diseases such as leukaemia there is the further need to destroy all remaining malignant cells. Centres specializing in bone marrow transplantation have gradually evolved methods of management, but there are still many problems even in the most experienced hands.

The preparation of the recipient involves intensive chemotherapy with high doses of cytotoxic drugs over a few days, plus in some cases total body irradiation.

A unit of blood is usually taken from the donor a week before the marrow donation and is given back afterwards. The bone marrow is removed by multiple marrow puncture, under spinal or general anaesthesia. This is followed by a few days of discomfort, but is only very rarely accompanied by any other disability. The donor marrow is put into a special fluid containing an anticoagulant and after filtration is injected into the blood stream of the recipient through a vein.

The next few weeks following the transplant, before signs that the graft has taken, are especially hazardous. Lack of white cells and suppression of immunity mean that the risk of infection is very high, and lack of platelets leads to risk of bleeding. The patient therefore needs to be isolated with fully available supportive treatment — transfusions of red cells, white cells, and platelets when indicated, and strict measures to prevent infection or to recognize and treat it if and when it occurs.

If the transplant takes signs of marrow regeneration appear in 2–4 weeks. As the white count rises the risks of infection are somewhat reduced, but immunity is impaired for many more months leaving the patient still susceptible to bacterial and viral infection.

There are other difficulties to be overcome. With increasing experience graft rejection has become less common, but is more likely to occur if a patient has had many transfusions before the transplant which may cause sensitization to antigens other than the HLA group. The recommendation now is, if a suitable donor is available, to transplant marrow to patients with severe aplastic anaemia as early as possible and preferably before any transfusions have been given.

Bone marrow transplantation

The next problem is graft-versus-host disease (GVHD). This is a condition which may occur early (within the first two or three months after the transplant) as an acute reaction or later in a chronic form. The disease is due to an immune reaction of donor lymphocytes against the recipient's tissues, and probably indicates a difference in minor histocompatibility antigens other than the HLA group.

In the acute form skin rashes, diarrhoea, and liver damage are the main symptoms and may prove fatal. In the more chronic form, which is seen in almost half the patients, a wide variety of symptoms is seen with a predominance of skin and mucous membrane damage, but almost any tissue may be involved. Chronic graft versus host disease is more common in older age groups. The outlook is poor in those in whom chronic GVHD follows an acute attack. Various drugs are now given after transplantation to reduce the incidence and severity of graft-versus-host disease and, if it does appear, treatment with corticosteroids and an immunosuppressive agent is given. GVHD delays recovery of immunity, so the time during which infectious complications are likely to arise is prolonged.

In addition to these problems some damage may result directly from the drugs and X-ray treatment given before transplantation. Chronic lung changes may occur and in older patients fertility may be affected. Patients treated before puberty, with chemotherapy only, develop normally, but the addition of total body irradiation may reduce the rate of growth and is likely to delay puberty and reduce fertility.

The two principal indications at the present time for bone marrow transplantation are severe aplastic anaemia and some acute leukaemias. In severe aplastic anaemia most patients now have a very good chance of recovery from the disease if they can be managed through the early hazards, and transplantation has become the treatment of choice if there is an available donor, particularly in younger patients, since the outlook otherwise is so poor.

Blood Disorders

In leukaemia, transplants were initially carried out only in terminally ill patients with relapse of their disease. In spite of this the results were sufficiently good to lead to the view that bone marrow transplant should be considered in acute non-lymphoblastic leukaemias in first remission when the clinical state is good, and in acute lymphoblastic leukaemias who have relapsed but are in a second or subsequent remission (see Chapter 12). The results are now very encouraging in terms of long-term survival although unfortunately leukaemia does recur in some patients in spite of the conditioning before transplant. This recurrence is sometimes seen in the transplant rather than the recipient cells, which suggests the possibility that a viral agent may be involved. Interestingly, long-term survival in remission is *improved* by the occurrence of some degree of graft-versus-host disease which appears to have some kind of antileukaemic effect.

Bone marrow transplantation is increasingly being considered for other diseases. Some patients with chronic granulocytic leukaemia (see Chapter 12) have been treated in this way and there is active interest, though as yet little experience, in the possible use in some patients with congenital red cell disorders, for example thalassaemia major (see Chapter 8). Bone marrow transplant has also been applied to some of the conditions where children are born with a deficiency in their immune system.

This is one of the expanding fields in medicine, but it must be emphasized that this treatment can only be carried out at special centres where all the necessary expertise and facilities are available.

14

Disorders of plasma cells

The subgroup of lymphocytes called B cells are concerned with the production of immune proteins or antibodies (immunoglobulins). Stimulation of B cells results in changes in the cells through various stages to a final one, the plasma cell. At any of these stages of stimulation, but particularly at the plasma cell stage, the cells manufacture and secrete immunoglobulins.

The whole B-cell system is not homogeneous. It is made up of several groups of cells each derived from a single stem cell, so that there are many different clones of B cells each of which produces a different immunoglobulin. In the group of disorders described in this chapter one clone predominates so that these conditions are characterized by the overproduction of a single type of immunoglobulin (monoclonal proliferation). This is in contrast to the normal situation when, for example, in response to a challenge from a bacterial infection a whole range of immunoglobulins will be produced (polyclonal proliferation).

The immunoglobulin molecules are made up of four chains of amino acids, two of which are called 'heavy chains' and two 'light chains'. These chains are manufactured separately within the cells and are assembled together only just before release from the cell. In some disorders incomplete immunoglobulin molecules may be produced, resulting in an excess of free light or heavy chains.

Various techniques can be used to demonstrate the proportion of different immunoglobulins in the plasma. If a drop of plasma is placed on absorbent paper, and an electric charge is passed through it, the different proteins will separate out in a recognizable pattern (protein electrophoresis). If one immunoglobulin is present in excess it will predominate and form a monoclonal, or M, band. The particular type of protein involved can be further defined by the use of antisera prepared against the different types of light and heavy chains.

Abnormal immunoglobulins (called paraproteins) may be produced in a number of conditions including some cases of chronic lymphatic leukaemia and lymphoma, but there are other disorders in which the primary abnormality is a malignant growth of a clone of immunoglobulin producing cells.

Myeloma

Myeloma is the most common malignant tumour of the plasma cells. It is very rare in young people, being a disease of later life with a peak incidence in the sixties and seventies. It is a slow-growing tumour and may take 15–20 years to produce symptoms. In some 10 per cent of cases the diagnosis is made by chance when an unexplained high erythrocyte sedimentation rate (ESR) is discovered. Laboratory tests may then reveal the presence of an abnormal pattern of immunoglobulins, and further investigations will confirm the diagnosis of myeloma.

There are two predominant features of the disease: first, symptoms due to infiltration of the bones by abnormal plasma cells; and second, involvement of the kidneys leading to kidney failure. General symptoms of tiredness, weakness and malaise are common, but in most patients the first symptom is bone pain, particularly in the ribs and back. This is caused by erosion which causes the bones to become weak and prone to fracture. Sudden onset of a severe pain without previous injury may indicate such a fracture in a rib, or collapse of one of the bones of the vertebral column (backbone). Even if there is no sudden fracture the softening of the bones may result in partial collapse of the vertebrae with consequent loss of height.

When the bone infiltration is widespread the destruction may produce a rise of the calcium in the blood to dangerous levels. This will cause depression, lack of appetite and vomiting, leading to dehydration and worsening of any kidney damage that may be present.

The kidney damage is the result of the overproduction of light chains, which is a feature of more than half the cases of myeloma. The light chains are filtered through the kidney where they tend to precipitate and cause an inflammatory reaction. The excretion of light chains in the urine (Bence Jones protein) is a diagnostic feature of myeloma but it is not found in all cases. The outlook is much worse in patients with serious kidney damage.

The level of the abnormal proteins in the plasma may be such that the blood becomes more viscous and circulation is impaired. But this is less common than in the condition of macroglobulinaemia described below. The sludging up of blood in small vessels caused by the hyperviscosity, may affect the blood-vessels in the brain causing impairment of mental function or vision. The paraproteins may also sometimes interfere with platelets or clotting factors, and this results in nose bleeds or bruising.

Occasionally a mass of myeloma tissue presses on the spinal cord and causes paralysis. If treated urgently the pressure can be relieved by operation on the spine and recovery of function may be good, but delay in treatment may result in irreversible damage to the spinal cord.

Normal immunoglobulin production is suppressed in myeloma, and patients are therefore prone to infections, particularly of the chest and urinary tract.

Once the condition of myeloma is suspected it is fairly easy to confirm the diagnosis. Examination of the blood usually shows a moderate anaemia. In the blood film the red cells are piled together (rouleaux), and the excess of abnormal protein is often shown as a bluish-staining background to the cells. The bone marrow shows either a patchy or diffuse infiltration with malignant plasma cells (Plate 13a) (in normal bone marrow only occasional plasma cells are found). The specific immunoglobulin type produced by the abnormal cells can be identified by special staining methods.

Further identification of the type of paraprotein involved in the disease is made by electrophoresis of the serum and the urine. The normal immunoglobulins are reduced or absent and a dominant peak, 'M band', is found in the serum. In the urine, excess light chains (Bence Jones protein) may be found.

The myeloma cells cause erosions which show up on X-ray examination of bones as punched-out translucent areas, particularly in the skull, ribs, pelvis and vertebrae (Plate 13b). Occasionally the tumours extend beyond the bones to give soft tissue masses.

Where the diagnosis is made by chance, and there is no sign of extensive bone involvement or kidney damage, there is no good evidence that active treatment is required, but careful follow up is necessary.

One of the most important recommendations is for patients to maintain a high fluid intake which helps to minimize any kidney damage. It is also vital to seek immediate medical attention for any intercurrent infection. Patients should remain as active as possible with the help of analgesics as required, since immobility only worsens the weakening of the bones. Localized areas of acute pain or tenderness may be treated with radiotherapy which often gives great symptomatic relief. Where there is anaemia blood transfusion may be indicated.

There are two main drugs, both nitrogen mustard derivatives, which are used in treatment of myeloma: melphelan and cyclophosphamide. The former, and more widely used, is sometimes combined with the steroid prednisolone and may be given in continuous low dosage or intermittently at a higher dose. The drugs are toxic, especially to the normal bone marrow, and treatment therefore requires careful medical supervision with regular blood counts and close cooperation between the patient and those involved in directing the treatment. In this disease, as in other neoplastic disorders, teams of doctors are constantly investigating ways of improving the outlook by variation in the drugs used, or the dose or method of administration.

Chemotherapy may reduce the tumour mass, with consequent reduction in paraprotein and general improvement in symptoms. Unfortunately, to date no cure has been achieved. The outlook depends largely on the severity of the disease at diagnosis, and particularly on the degree of kidney involvement. Sooner or later the condition is likely to escape from control, and deteriorating kidney function, infection, or in occasional cases a transformation to a form of leukaemia, will lead to death.

Waldenström's macroglobulinaemia

Waldenström is a Swedish physician who first described the features of this condition in 1944. Like myeloma it is a disease of elderly people but differs in that it mainly affects men.

The onset of symptoms is insidious with general complaints of lassitude, weakness and weight loss. Other symptoms are largely determined by the particular type of paraprotein, called a macroglobulin, which is produced in excess. The macroglobulin is responsible for a striking increase in the viscosity of the blood resulting in visual disturbances, bleeding into the retina (the light-sensitive layer at the back of the eye), and mental changes of confusion, lack of concentration, or clouding of consciousness. The tendency to bleed is more frequent than in myeloma, and nose bleeds and purpura (a rash caused by rupture of small capillaries in the skin) are common. Sometimes there is weakness or numbness in one or more limbs, due to involvement of the peripheral nerves. The causal relationship between these symptoms and the macroglobulin is not known for certain.

The macroglobulin may also be a cryoglobulin, that is one which comes out of solution in the cold or even at room temperature causing obstruction to the circulation of blood in exposed areas such as the hands, nose and ears. Occasionally small vessels may be completely blocked with consequent loss of tissue. Infection is not so great a problem as in myeloma since the normal immunoglobulins are not as a rule so severely depressed.

A moderate degree of lymph node enlargement may be present, and the spleen and liver may also be enlarged.

Anaemia is common, and although the white count is seldom increased there is usually some increase in the proportion of lymphocytes. There may be difficulty in making a blood count and spreading a blood film because of the tendency of the cells to pile up together (rouleaux formation). Sometimes the plasma of the sample gels or forms a precipitate at room temperature. As in myeloma the blood film may show a bluish background staining of the paraprotein. The bone marrow is often somewhat hypocellular but shows an increase in lymphoid and plasma cells, which with special staining can be shown to be producing the abnormal type of protein. Confirmation of the diagnosis is by the identification of the macroglobulin in the serum.

It is doubtful whether any specific treatment alters the outlook in this condition, although a variety of drugs has been used including the nitrogen mustard derivatives melphelan, cyclophosphamide and chlorambucil. On the other hand, where symptoms of obstruction to the blood circulation are related to the mass of abnormal protein these may be relieved by removing the bulk of the patient's own plasma, and at the same time replacing it with normal plasma (plasmapheresis). The red cells are separated during this process so that they can be returned to the patient's circulation. Symptomatic relief may last for some time as regeneration of the abnormal protein is often quite slow. The process can be repeated when indicated.

Disorders of plasma cells

Benign paraproteinaemia

This is a condition which, as its name implies, produces no symptoms. It is usually found only by chance when, during investigation of some other complaint, the erythrocyte sedimentation rate (ESR) is found to be unusually high. The incidence increases with age and it is found in about 3 per cent of healthy people over the age of 70 years. The importance of the condition lies in the fact that it may be confused with more serious disorders of the plasma cells. Sometimes it is indeed difficult to say whether the finding of the paraprotein indicates an early phase in the development of an underlying malignancy, particularly of the lymphoid system, but the fact that the level of the paraprotein remains stable over a long period of observation, that normal immunoglobulins are not suppressed, and that there is only a small excess of plasma cells in the bone marrow are all indications that the condition is benign.

15

Malignant disorders of lymph glands

Lymph is a fluid which is drained from the tissues through fine tubes called lymphatics. At intervals along the lymphatics there are small swellings or nodes — the lymph nodes — which occur in groups in sites such as the armpit or groin. Lymphoma is the term used for a malignant condition of the lymph nodes which also may involve other organs where lymphoid tissue is found such as the spleen, liver, bone marrow, and gut. Two broad groups are recognized: Hodgkin's disease, and the so-called non-Hodgkin lymphomas.

The causes of the lymphomas are probably multiple. Although from time to time clusters of Hodgkin's disease have been reported, it is doubtful if these are of significance and no real clue as to the cause of Hodgkin's disease has emerged.

In the case of non Hodgkin lymphomas, there has been renewed interest in the possible role of viruses since the finding that the Epstein-Barr (EB) virus (the cause of glandular fever) is closely associated with a type of lymphoma called Burkitt's lymphoma, which occurs particularly in East Africa and Papua New Guinea. An additional factor seems to be necessary to induce the lymphoma, and it has been suggested that this might be malaria since the areas where the tumour is prevalent are also those in which malaria is common. Genetic factors could also be involved.

The HTLV virus (human T cell leukaemia virus) has been found in certain types of lymphoma as well as leukaemia, where the origin of the tumour cells is from the subtype of lymphocytes called T cells, but the search for viruses in other types of lymphoma has so far been negative.

As with leukaemias one factor for predisposition to the

Malignant disorders of lymph glands

development of lymphoma is any form of deficiency in the immune system, such as occurs in the congenital immune deficiency syndromes and following immunosuppressive treatment, or in diseases such as rheumatoid arthritis in which autoimmunity plays a part.

Such possible clues as to the cause are, however, found in only a small minority of lymphomas. In most cases no predisposing factors can be identified.

Hodgkin's disease

The physician who first described cases of this disease in 1832 was Thomas Hodgkin of Guy's Hospital. He had observed seven patients, all of whom died, with enlargement of lymph glands and spleen. Some 60–70 years later the characteristics of the microscopical appearances of the abnormal glands were described, and these still form the basis for the diagnosis of Hodgkin's disease.

The disease has two peaks of incidence, in young adults and in an over-55 age group, and is more common in men than women. Usually the first symptom noted is painless enlargement of one or more lymph nodes, most commonly in the neck or armpit, much less frequently in the groin. Sometimes enlarged glands are first discovered in the chest during a routine X-ray examination. There may be no other symptoms or there may be some weight loss, fever causing heavy sweats at night, or skin itching. This last symptom may precede the appearance of any gland enlargement. A striking but rare symptom is pain in the glands induced by drinking alcohol.

Hodgkin's disease, and indeed all lymphomas, have to be distinguished from other conditions which cause swelling of lymph nodes. Many conditions, such as glandular fever, German measles, or septic infections can be ruled out on the basis of the history, and blood or bacteriological tests. Often, however, the diagnosis is not obvious and removal of a gland for microscopical examination is essential (lymph node biopsy). In Hodgkin's disease, as well as making the diagnosis on sections of the lymph node, the pathologist can distinguish four different varieties which have a bearing on the response to treatment.

In the old days, without specific treatment about half the patients died within a year of diagnosis, and less then 10 per cent survived as long as five years. Early forms of X-ray treatment produced some improvement but relapse of the disease was the rule. In those pioneering days there were no reliable methods for measuring the dose of X-rays and in the light of modern treatment the management was crude. Since the 1920s progressive developments in radiotherapy have led to far more precise and effective treatment. Parallel with this there have been great advances in the use of chemical agents (chemotherapy), so that far from being a fatal illness, Hodgkin's disease is now curable in a high proportion of cases.

In order to choose the most appropriate treatment it is necessary to define the extent of the disease as precisely as possible. Hodgkin's disease is believed to arise in one group of glands and then spread to glands in adjacent areas, eventually becoming widespread throughout the body. The process of defining the extent of the disease is called 'staging'.

There are four separate stages. In the earliest stage, stage 1, the disease is confined to one group of nodes, for example on one side of the neck. In stage II, more than one site is involved but on the same side of the diaphragm (the muscle which divides the chest from the abdomen). In stage III, there is evidence of disease both above and below the diaphragm, and in stage IV there is widespread disease involving sites other than lymph nodes, for example liver, bone marrow or skin. In staging, a note is made of whether or not there has been weight loss and/or fever (described as B symptoms) for these usually indicate more advanced disease.

Several investigations — including a blood count and biochemical tests, bone marrow examination, and a chest X-ray — are needed to determine the staging. In order to study glands in the pelvis and abdomen a special X-ray called a lymphogram (or lymphangiogram) is used. A radio-opaque dye is injected into a lymphatic vessel in each foot. The dye travels upwards and fills the lymph nodes which then show up on X-ray. Involved lymph nodes have an abnormal foamy appearance. A kidney X-ray is also required as this may show displacement of the ureters (the tubes connecting the kidneys and bladder) by abdominal glands which have not been shown up by the lymphangiogram. Whole body scanners, now gradually becoming more widely available, can be of great assistance in defining enlarged glands, and are increasingly used in preference to lymphangiograms.

The final investigation, which sounds alarming to the patient whose only complaint may be of a painless swelling in the neck or armpit, is a 'staging laparotomy'. This means that when all the other tests indicate a stage 1, II, or IIIA disease an abdominal operation may be recommended, to search carefully for any other glands which may be involved, but have remained undetected, and at the same time to remove the spleen since it is sometimes involved even when not enlarged. Laparotomy increases the staging in a considerable proportion of cases, but in about 3–10 per cent glands which were thought to be abnormal on lymphangiogram prove to be normal.

In the hands of an experienced team the operation gives remarkably little trouble. Recently, however, the necessity for laparotomy has been questioned in some centres since it is agreed that if a relapse occurs from an undisclosed site, it can be controlled by further treatment. On the other hand, in patients in whom staging is reduced by laparotomy treatment can be more limited.

In the rare cases of Hodgkin's disease in childhood staging laparotomy is generally not advised, first, because removal of the spleen predisposes to severe infections in children, and second, because X-ray treatment may have detrimental effects

131

on growth and development and therefore may not be the first choice in children. These are still controversial problems.

After full investigation, apart from young children, those who are classed as stage I or II disease are treated by radiotherapy. Stage IV patients are always given chemotherapy, and stage III patients may be given chemotherapy or radiotherapy, depending on precisely which lymph nodes are involved and whether there are any 'B symptoms'. If such symptoms are present the treatment of choice is chemotherapy. Some centres are now attempting to improve results by combining radiotherapy and chemotherapy.

Because of the way Hodgkin's disease spreads from one group of glands to adjacent groups, radiotherapy is planned to include not only the primary site but all other nearby groups of glands. The course usually lasts about 6–8 weeks with treatment on 5 days a week, but this may need to be modified according to the effects on the blood.

The earliest successful chemotherapy was with single drugs, many of which proved of temporary benefit, but usually at the expense of considerable toxicity. It was argued that a combination of drugs, each with different toxic effects, could be given in lower dosage which might reduce the overall toxicity but enhance the overall benefit. This in fact proved to be the case. Several combinations have been used, but most include an alkalating agent (nitrogen mustard, or chlorambucil), one of the vinca-alkaloids (vincristine or vinblastine), a corticosteroid (predisolone), and another agent called procarbazine.

The drugs are usually given in two-week courses with an interval of 2–4 weeks between to allow the bone marrow to recover. Some depression of white cells and platelets often occurs, and the courses may need to be adjusted accordingly by reducing the doses of drugs or prolonging the interval between courses. About six courses in all are given, unless the disease is unusually resistant when longer treatment may be needed. Most patients, however, respond quickly and rapidly become symptom-free and able to lead a normal and active

Malignant disorders of lymph glands

life. Indeed, many need strong encouragement to keep up the treatment since they justifiably claim that the only time they feel ill is during treatment! This is particularly so with injections of nitrogen mustard which produce nausea and vomiting, but if these symptoms are unbearable a change can be made to chlorambucil (an oral and less toxic nitrogen mustard-like drug).

Temporary loss of hair may occur with the use of vincristine, and some patients develop tingling or pains in the legs or jaw which may be sufficiently troublesome to need a switch to the similar drug vinblastine, which, however, has the disadvantage of being more toxic to the bone marrow.

Fertility is likely to be affected by the drug treatment, particularly in young men, and most young women stop menstruating. Recent studies, however, suggest that recovery of fertility may occur in some cases, especially in women. The possibility of storing sperm before the start of treatment for future artificial insemination can be considered for those young men who fear a loss of fertility.

Hodgkin's disease is one of the conditions in which immunity is impaired, and this is exaggerated by chemotherapy. This means that intercurrent infections may be a serious problem — shingles (herpes zoster), for instance is a very frequent complication and requires prompt treatment with antiviral agents.

With modern treatment about 90 per cent of patients with stage I and II disease, 70–80 per cent of stage III patients, and about 60 per cent of stage IV patients are alive at five years after diagnosis, although some from each stage will have relapsed. Such recurrence, however, may respond well to further treatment. In all groups, those who have been in continuous remission for five years are likely to have been cured.

One long-term effect which is seen in some patients is the development of second malignancies, particularly non-Hodgkin lymphomas and leukaemia. The incidence may be of the order of one to two per 1000 patients. At the present time there seems no way of avoiding this possible hazard although, as in leukaemia, special centres are continually involved in reviewing treatment and attempting to improve the outlook still further.

Non-Hodgkin lymphomas

The term non-Hodgkin lymphoma includes a great variety of conditions which have in common uncontrolled growth of lymphoid tissue. Unlike Hodgkin's disease, these lymphomas tend to originate in more than one site and to spread diffusely through lymphoid tissue, with a particular tendency to involve the bone marrow.

Non-Hodgkin lymphomas are relatively uncommon under the age of 40, and have a peak incidence between 55 and 70 years of age. Unlike Hodgkin's disease there is little difference in sex incidence. In many patients the initial clinical picture is similar to Hodgkin's disease and can only be distinguished by lymph node biopsy (see p. 129). Pathologists distinguish two main groups: low-grade lymphomas with 'good histology', and high-grade lymphomas with 'bad histology'. In low-grade lymphomas the evolution and progress of the disorder may be very slow, often with intervals when the enlarged glands seem to disappear. In the high-grade lymphomas the disease is more aggressive and the outlook poorer. Classification of the different types of lymphoma included in these two main groups is still a matter for discussion among pathologists, as more techniques are developed for distinguishing the origin of different types of cells.

About a third of the patients, when first seen, have infiltration of organs outside the lymph nodes, particularly in the skin, bone marrow and gut. Lymphoma developing first in the gut is particularly common in Middle Eastern peoples. It may be brought to light as the result of intestinal bleeding or obstructive symptoms, and be diagnosed only at operation.

Unless the bone marrow or spleen are involved the

Malignant disorders of lymph glands

lymphomas may produce little or no disturbance of the blood, but when they are invaded anaemia, neutropenia or depression of platelets may be seen. Sometimes an autoimmune haemolytic anaemia or thrombocytopenia (lack of platelets) develops which may respond to corticosteroid treatment, or may require removal of the spleen.

Investigation and staging of the disease is similar to that for Hodgkin's disease, but staging laparotomy is no longer recommended. The operation is not so well tolerated in the older age group, and in any event 60–80 per cent of patients already have evidence of spread to other sites at diagnosis.

The presence or absence of 'B symptoms' is very important in gauging the probable outlook. In all types of lymphoma B symptoms are an unfavourable sign. Many patients who have one of the low-grade lymphomas, and no B symptoms, are often just kept under observation and may require no treatment for years. In some of these, spontaneous improvement may occur for a time. Others have troublesome enlargement of glands which can be reduced in size by radiotherapy localized to the involved nodes. Many of the patients are elderly, and are less disturbed by such treatment than by attempting a 'cure' with aggressive chemotherapy. If their condition appears to be progressive, relatively mild chemotherapy with chlorambucil with or without prednisolone may bring it under control. More aggressive regimes have no advantage in such patients. On the other hand, the high-grade lymphomas, especially when associated with B symptoms, have a poor outlook if untreated, and various schedules of chemotherapy using three or more drugs (combination chemotherapy) are used in such cases, unless the disease appears limited when X-ray treatment may be considered. Even then radiation is usually followed by chemotherapy.

The types of regime used for treatment of the high-grade lymphomas often prove very toxic to such patients who are so frequently elderly, and the possible benefits have to be weighed up carefully against the discomforts and complica-

135

tions of treatment. Nevertheless if remission can be achieved there is a possibility of prolonged disease-free survival.

As in other malignant blood disorders supportive care is extremely important. There is a constant danger of inter-current infections, particularly chest infections, and shingles is a frequent complication, as in Hodgkin's disease.

16

Abnormal bleeding

Although the blood in circulation is fluid, a wound does not normally bleed for more than a few minutes unless a major artery is involved. The arrest of bleeding is called haemostasis. The process is amazingly complex, and involves reactions of the blood-vessels to injury, alterations in the platelets, and the interaction of a whole series of factors in the plasma leading finally to the formation of a blood clot (blood coagulation). Disorders characterized by an abnormal tendency to bleed may be associated with defects in any of the many steps involved.

Blood clotting

The sequence of events following an injury is: first, the severed blood-vessel contracts. Then the platelets stick to the damaged lining of the vessel and pile up to form a 'haemostatic plug'. These processes are called platelet 'adhesion' and 'aggregation', and they are defective in some blood disorders.

While the haemostatic plug is forming the reactions leading to clotting of the blood are set in train. The platelets are one of the trigger factors, but components of the damaged vessel wall also play an important role in starting off the process which has been likened to a cascade or waterfall. It involves twelve recognized factors. Each of these is normally present in an inert form, but once the chain of reactions has been triggered they are each activated in turn by their preceding factor. The final step is the conversion of the soluble plasma protein called fibrinogen, to strands of an insoluble protein, called fibrin, which makes up the framework of the clot and in which are trapped red cells, white cells and platelets. The clot then shrinks, squeezing out any plasma which has also been trapped. The shrinking is caused by the platelets, 'clot retraction' being another important function of these small but complex elements.

During the clotting process an opposing system is called into action. This is called fibrinolysis, and it is responsible for clearing up the debris of a clot once bleeding has been stopped.

Understanding of all the complexities of blood coagulation has been achieved largely through the study of rare blood disorders, in which absence of one or other of the clotting factors is responsible for a bleeding tendency. It may well be that the story is still incomplete.

Bleeding disorders due to platelet abnormalities

Abnormalities of platelets lead to failure of the early stage of haemostasis, and lack of formation of a haemostatic plug. This leads to immediate and prolonged bleeding after injury. In addition, platelets are concerned with keeping the lining of blood-vessels intact. The lining cells (endothelial cells) are constantly being shed and renewed, and the platelets help to 'stop the gaps'. If they fail to do so, leaking tends to occur very easily from small vessels even without obvious injury, particularly under the skin and in the mucous membranes. This is shown by symptoms such as bruising, petechiae (tiny bleeding points under the skin), blood blisters in the mouth, bleeding from the gums, nose-bleeds, and heavy menstrual periods.

The characteristic laboratory finding is of a prolonged 'bleeding time'. The simplest way to measure this is to make a small puncture in an ear lobe, and to touch the drop of blood with absorbent paper every half-minute. The time taken to stop bleeding is normally less than 3 minutes. Another method is more standardized, and involves making a very small incision in the forearm to a depth of exactly 3 mm after a blood pressure cuff has been put on the arm and pumped up to a standard pressure. The average bleeding time from three cuts should be not more than four minutes. In severe platelet deficiencies bleeding may continue for very much longer, and will have to be stopped by applying pressure.

Platelets may be deficient in number (thrombocytopenia) or functionally abnormal.

Bleeding does not usually occur until the platelet count is quite low — about a tenth of the normal level. In some conditions the count may be close to zero and the danger of bleeding is then severe.

A low platelet count is a feature of many blood disorders such as megaloblastic anaemia, leukaemia, or aplastic anaemia. It is also one of the commonest types of adverse reaction to drugs. This may be due to an immune reaction comparable with that seen in some cases of drug-induced haemolytic anaemia and agranulocytosis (see pp. 67, 94), or to a suppression of platelet formation. Many drugs may occasionally cause thrombocytopenia. When this is due to an immune response the onset of symptoms is usually acute and occurs after reintroduction of a drug which has been taken previously. Drugs that suppress formation of platelets produce a more gradual onset of symptoms; often the depression may be part of a more general effect on the bone marrow.

The drug most frequently associated with immune thrombocytopenia is quinine. It is not always realized that quinine may be a component of some proprietary preparations that can be bought over the counter; Anadin is one such example, which in a sensitized individual can cause acute thrombocytopenia. The quinine in tonic water or other bitter soft drinks can also cause trouble. Most cases of drug-induced thrombocytopenia will recover quickly when the offending agent is withdrawn, but where bone marrow suppression is the cause the recovery may take somewhat longer.

Another form of thrombocytopenia goes under the names of 'idiopathic thrombocytopenic purpura' (ITP), 'primary thrombocytopenia' or 'autoimmine thrombocytopenia'. As

139

the last name implies it is caused by an autoimmune response, with the production of antibodies which destroy the platelets, the condition being comparable to autoimmune haemolytic anaemia (see Chapter 7).

Idiopathic thrombocytopenic purpura occurs in an acute and chronic or intermittent form. The acute form affects mainly children and occurs equally in boys and girls. It is usually preceded by a few days to about 3 weeks by an obvious viral infection, particularly German measles and influenza. In nearly every case the disorder recovers spontaneously within a few weeks, but recovery may be hastened by a short course of corticosteroids.

Adults tend to have an intermittent or chronic course to idiopathic thrombocytopenic purpura, and the condition is three to four times more common in women than men. Evidence that the condition is due to an autoimmune reaction came in 1951 when workers in St Louis, United States, showed that plasma from patients with ITP produced a fall in platelets when injected into normal volunteers, and concluded that the thrombocytopenic factor was a platelet antibody. The antibody is able to pass through the placenta so that babies born to mothers with ITP have neonatal thrombocytopenia, which recovers as the antibody gradually disappears.

The diagnosis of ITP depends on the history, evidence of bleeding characteristic of a platelet defect, the finding of a low platelet count, and elimination of other causes for a low platelet count. The bone marrow is usually active, and mega-karyocytes (the early platelet forming cells) are often increased in number. The spleen is not enlarged, a feature which helps to distinguish this disease from thrombocytopenia secondary to other conditions.

Corticosteroids produce a rise in platelets and arrest of bleeding in the majority of patients, but most will relapse when the steroids are stopped. The most effective treatment is removal of the spleen, which produces lasting improvement in almost all cases. Unfortunately it is impossible to predict which may be the few failures, but those who do fail to respond to operation may be kept free of symptoms by a small dose of steroids. Failing that, immunosuppressive drugs such as azathioprine or cyclophosphamide may be tried.

Occasionally, failure to respond to splenectomy, or recurrence of thrombocytopenia after an initial good response, can be attributed to the presence of an 'accessory' spleen. There are often small bits of splenic tissue in addition to the main organ, and these, if not removed at operation, can take over splenic function and cause a relapse in the thrombocytopenia. They can sometimes be identified by special radiological techniques.

Some patients with a chronic course may have little trouble, although intercurrent infections may cause a temporary lowering of the platelet count. They may be better managed by intermittent treatment with steroids when indicated by the symptoms, rather than submitted to an operation.

The occasional development of an immune thrombocytopenia in the course of other diseases such as a lymphoma may respond to treatment by splenectomy if not controlled by treatment of the underlying disorder. If the spleen is much enlarged an alternative cause of thrombocytopenia may be 'pooling' of platelets in the spleen thus removing them from circulation. Splenectomy is also often beneficial in this situation.

There are a number of inherited disorders of platelets which result in a lifelong tendency to bleeding. The clinical picture is similar to that in thrombocytopenia but the platelet count is normal. Tests of platelet function, however, such as the bleeding time, and ability of the platelets to aggregate, show them to be functionally defective. These conditions are inherited as recessive characters (see Chapter 3). The severity is very variable and there is no specific treatment. Women who have severe menstrual bleeding may need hormone treatment to suppress ovulation.

Blood Disorders

Disorders due to coagulation defects

Bleeding associated with an abnormality in one of the clotting factors differs from that due to platelet defects, in that the initial stages of haemostasis (contraction of vessels and formation of the platelet plug) are normal so that bleeding does not occur immediately after injury but is delayed. A further feature is that bleeding tends to be into deeper tissues, for example muscles and joints, and may be not be unusual from pricks or superficial abrasions.

Only three of the many defects of coagulation are relatively common. These are haemophilia, Christmas disease (named after the person first identified as having this disorder) and von Willebrand's disease. The first two have a similar clinical picture and can be distinguished only in the laboratory.

Haemophilia and Christmas disease

These two are caused by an abnormal sex-linked gene carried on the X chromosome (see chapter 3) and therefore only occuring in males. The most notable carrier was Queen Victoria, two of whose daughters, Alice and Beatrice, were carriers and one son, Leopold, suffered from haemophilia. The family tree shows the classical type of inheritance of an X-linked disorder. Victoria's daughter Alice had a haemophiliac son and two carrier daughters, one of whom, Alix, married Czar Nicholas of Russia. The sinister presence of Rasputin in the Russian court was associated with his supposed influence on the bleeding episodes of their haemophiliac son Alexei. The gene appears to have died out in the fifth generation and there is now no means of knowing whether the disorder was classical haemophilia or Christmas disease.

Haemophilia is caused by a deficiency of part of the protein in plasma called antihaemophiliac globulin or factor VIII. In Christmas disease the deficiency is in a different factor, factor IX. The severity of these diseases is variable but tends to follow the same pattern within families. Abnormal bruising or

Abnormal bleeding

bleeding is usually first recognized at circumcision, or later when the child starts to move around actively. Then mild or unnoticed trauma produces large lumpy bruises or bleeding into muscles and joints which is very painful. There is sometimes blood in the urine or bleeding from the bowel. Bleeding in the mouth may be particularly dangerous if blood tracks down into the neck where it may obstruct the airway. Uncontrolled bleeding into muscles may cause pressure on nerves or develop into large blood cysts. Repeated bleeding into joints causes destructive changes which result in permanent damage and limitation of movement.

Fortunately all these symptoms may now be greatly modified by treatment with preparations of the missing factors VIII or IX. Many patients can now lead more normal lives with the supervision and support given by special centres. Indeed with good control life expectancy is near normal. At many centres home treatment is now encouraged. The patient or one of his family is taught to inject the missing factor into a vein; many patients come to recognize the first signs of trouble and can give treatment in time to prevent a serious episode.

Dental extractions which used to be followed by prolonged and sometimes dangerous bleeding, and any other surgical procedures, can now be safely undertaken under supervision and administration of sufficient of the missing factor to control bleeding. With such modern management these previously severe and crippling diseases, often with early mortality, can usually be reasonably controlled and much suffering avoided.

Unfortunately, a few patients develop antibodies to the factors used in treatment. This creates great difficulties and attempts to suppress the antibody with immunosuppressant drugs have been disappointing.

Another risk from treatment is the development of hepatitis (a liver infection caused by a virus). Even if blood donors are screened for evidence of previous hepatitis not all types of the virus can be detected, and the infection can be transmitted in plasma products. Another more worrying feature is the recent recognition of the occurrence of AIDS (acquired immune deficiency syndrome) in a few haemophiliacs. The incidence is probably of the order of 0.8 per 1000 haemophiliacs. Recent evidence indicates that a virus similar but not identical to the human T-cell leukaemia virus (HTLV III) is responsible. Haemophilia centres, and manufacturers of plasma products, are actively pursuing possible methods for reducing the risks of treatment. The most effective approach promises to be through the artificial production of antihaemophilic globulin by genetic engineering.

Genetic counselling plays an important role in the management of patients with haemophilia and Christmas disease. Men with these disorders should realize that all their sons will be normal but all their daughters will be carriers. A proportion of carriers can be identified by measurement of the relevant factors in their blood, but some carriers have findings within the normal range so identification cannot be certain.

Antenatal diagnosis of the sex of a fetus is possible, and termination of pregnancy with a male fetus may be contemplated on the basis that there is an equal chance of the child being normal or affected, but fortunately advances in technology are making it more possible for the positive detection of haemophilia prenatally.

Von Willebrand's disease

A familial bleeding disorder which occurred in both sexes was described in 1926 by a Swedish physician, von Willebrand, as pseudohaemophilia. The disease has features both of a platelet abnormality and a coagulation defect. There are two genetic types: in one the inheritance is by an autosomal dominant gene; in the other more severe and rarer form, as an autosomal recessive, the parents of such cases often being blood relatives.

In the more common form the first symptoms are usually bruising and bleeding from mucous membranes, for example

144

nosebleeds. Heavy menstrual periods are common. In the more severe form the picture is more like haemophilia. Laboratory diagnosis depends on finding a long bleeding time, plus defects in factor VIII formation.

Treatment is largely confined to the use of factor VIII preparations for severe episodes or before dental treatment or surgery. Heavy menstrual periods are often a major problem and may be severe enough to require removal of the womb.

Vitamin K deficiency

Some of the coagulation factors require vitamin K for their manufacture by the liver. This vitamin was discovered by a Danish investigator Henrik Dam. He had found that chicks fed a fat-free diet became anaemic and had a tendency to bleed, and later he showed that the bleeding could be prevented by a factor in cereals and seeds which he called 'Koagulations Vitamin' (vitamin K). The chemical structure and synthesis was achieved some years later.

In addition to its presence in food vitamin K is manufactured by bacteria in the gut. It is a fat-soluble vitamin and needs the presence of bile salts to be absorbed. In conditions where the flow of bile from the liver through the bile ducts into the intestine is obstructed by a gallstone or a tumour, a deficiency of vitamin K develops with resulting failure in production of the vitamin K-dependent clotting factors which in turn gives rise to bleeding. A similar picture results if the liver cells are damaged and are unable to manufacture clotting factors.

Haemorrhagic disease of the newborn

In this condition persistent bleeding occurs within the first week of life from the umbilicus, or as the result of any injury, or in the urine or faeces. The condition sometimes used to recover by itself, but early in this century it was found that transfusion rapidly cured the bleeding tendency. We now know that the beneficial effect of transfusion was due to supply of vitamin K-dependent clotting factors which are deficient in the newborn with haemorrhagic disease.

The discovery of vitamin K led to its application in treatment of this condition. The dose of vitamin K must be low, as the immature liver cannot deal with high doses and a haemolytic anaemia may occur as a complication. Severe cases of haemorrhagic disease may require transfusion with plasma containing the clotting factors, since the response to vitamin K may be delayed for 12 hours or more. The tendency to spontaneous recovery has been attributed to the commencement of feeding and to the colonization of the infant's gut by bacteria which manufacture vitamin K.

Oral anticoagulants

Oral anticoagulants are now widely used in the treatment of individuals who have developed a blockage of a blood-vessel by a clot (thrombosis).

They act by antagonizing vitamin K, and so reduce the production of the vitamin K-dependent clotting factors. The dosage of the anticoagulants has to be adjusted to that which will reduce the tendency to thrombosis, but will not produce bleeding. Stabilization may be difficult, especially when any other drugs are being used. Some drugs may enhance the effect of anticoagulants, others decrease the sensitivity. It is therefore important that once the effective dose has been found other drugs should not be changed except under supervision. Many centres have 'anticoagulant clinics' where the blood clotting may be regularly reviewed, and dosage adjusted as necessary.

Allergic purpura

This condition (also called Henoch-Schönlein disease) has been recognized since the middle of the last century, and is thought to be due to an allergic response to a variety of stimuli. It affects children principally and is rather more common in boys than girls. It is sometimes preceded by about 1–3 weeks by an infection, but it may also be induced by a food or drug allergy. In many cases no precipitating factor can be identified.

The onset is sudden and is characterized by a purpuric rash with a typical distribution over the buttocks and backs of the arms and legs (Plate 14). In addition there are often painful swellings round the joints and patches of oedema (localized collections of fluid under the skin). Similar oedematous areas in the bowel give rise to colicky abdominal pain sometimes accompanied by bleeding from the bowel. The kidneys are sometimes involved, and blood may appear in the urine.

The underlying lesion is an inflammatory reaction in small blood vessels (vasculitis). The platelet count and platelet function tests are normal. The white cell count may be raised, and the eosinophil granulocytes are sometimes increased. The diagnosis is made largely on the typical clinical picture.

The condition usually comes and goes for a few weeks and then disappears by itself, but if the kidneys are badly affected there may be some chronic kidney damage.

Easy bruising syndromes

Many women bruise easily, but are otherwise entirely healthy, and all available tests for abnormalities of platelets or clotting factors are normal. Occasionally this easy bruising is exploited in psychologically disturbed young women who are able to produce widespread purpuric lesions by self-inflicted trauma.

Another curious condition is apparently related to sensitivity of the patient (almost always a woman) to her own red cells (autoerythrocyte sensitization). The woman complains of sudden stinging pain, usually on an arm or leg, followed by the development of a raised red patch which gradually develops into a large painful bruise. A similar lesion can be produced by the injection of 0.1 ml of her own red cells under the skin. No such reaction is found in normal individuals. The condition comes and goes over a period of time, but tends eventually to disappear. Many of the individuals with this disorder are emotionally disturbed, and it is usually regarded as a psychosomatic illness.

Bleeding associated with vascular abnormalities

Blood vessels are normally supported by surrounding tissue containing fibres of a protein called collagen. In some conditions this supporting tissue is defective and small blood-vessels are liable to rupture.

The commonest example of such a state is the so-called 'senile purpura' of elderly people. As part of the ageing process the skin and underlying tissues become atrophic, and minor injuries result in escape of blood under the skin. This blood is absorbed slowly so that irregular dark purplish areas appear, particularly on the backs of the hands and on the forearms. Long-term treatment with corticosteroids may result in similar atrophic changes resulting in purpura.

Collagen is defective also in vitamin C deficiency (scurvy) and this results in extensive bruising and bleeding. In the infant fed boiled milk without any vitamin supplements bleeding from lack of vitamin C tends to occur under the layer of connective tissue overlying the bones (periosteum). In adults there may be bleeding into muscles and extensive bruising. Tiny haemorrhages are also seen at the base of the hairs, particularly on the legs (perifollicular haemorrhages). The gums, if there are teeth still present, become spongy and bleed easily. Scurvy is now seen mainly in elderly people, particularly old men living alone in poor circumstances on a diet lacking fresh fruit and vegetables, and it is readily treated with vitamin C (ascorbic acid).

There are a number of inherited disorders of collagen which are associated with a bleeding tendency. The defects affect the walls of the blood-vessels as well as the supporting tissue, so that bleeding from larger blood-vessels may occur, for example from the vessels in the walls of the gastrointestinal tract. Some of these disorders can be recognized by the paper-thin scars at the site of any injury, the abnormal 'stretchiness' of the skin, and hyperextensibility of the joints ('double joints').

Another fairly common inherited disorder associated with bleeding is hereditary haemorrhagic telangiectasia, also known as Osler–Weber–Rendu disease after the physicians who described the condition. The characteristic defect (telangiectasis) is the result of thinning of the walls of small veins and capillaries, which become dilated and tortuous and form blebs filled with blood which can be emptied by pressure. Sometimes there are only a few lesions visible on the lips or in the mouth but they may be widespread (Plate 15). Telangiectases may also occur in the gut, the air passages or genitourinary tract. Bleeding may arise from any of these sites, but by far the commonest symptom is recurrent nose bleeding. The lesions increase and become more obvious with age, which accounts for the fact that although the condition is hereditary (an autosomal dominant trait) symptoms of bleeding seldom occur until adult life.

Treatment consists mainly of local measures to stop the bleeding. If it has been severe and recurrent an iron deficiency anaemia may develop and need treatment. Bleeding from a lesion in the gut is often very difficult to locate and, since such lesions may be multiple, very difficult to deal with. Blood transfusion may be the only means of combating the anaemia.

17

The spleen

Mention has been made in previous chapters of the usefulness of splenectomy in alleviating some blood disorders. When advised to have this operation patients may wonder how they can do without a spleen, and what are its functions. The spleen is situated in the upper left-hand side of the abdominal cavity, behind the ribs and under the diaphragm, and cannot normally be felt on examination of the abdomen. It is a very vascular organ with a complex filtration system through which the blood flows. It contains a notably high concentration of macrophages (scavenging cells) and is therefore an important part of the reticuloendothelial system. It is also one of the major lymphatic organs.

In many animals the spleen acts as a reservoir of red cells which can rapidly be brought into circulation by contraction of the organ at times of aggression or exercise. In man this function is vestigial; the normal human spleen weighs only about 150 g and contains a mere 20–40 ml of blood, an insignificant amount compared with the total blood volume of some 4–5 litres.

During fetal life the spleen contains haemopoietic cells (red cell and white cell precursors). This 'extramedullary haemopoiesis' can reappear in some blood disorders when the blood production has become so much increased that it extends beyond the confines of the bones to other tissues, or when the bone marrow is replaced by fibrosis.

The main functions of the spleen are, however, to remove wornout or defective cells from the circulation and to assist in the immune defences of the body. Although in the first of these the spleen may play a major role, the reticuloendothelial cells elsewhere in the body can take on this function when the

The spleen

spleen is removed. One may wonder, therefore, why removal of the spleen is so effective in treating some conditions where the red cells are abnormal.

One reason is the fact that the minimal width of the channels through which red cells have to travel is less in the spleen than elsewhere in the body, and any factor which increases the rigidity or decreases the ability of the cells' to change shape in order to squeeze through narrow spaces will make them more likely to be trapped in the spleen than elsewhere, and subsequently removed by the macrophages (scavenging cells). In addition a proportion of the blood passing through the spleen circulates very slowly, and this produces local conditions which make destruction of abnormal cells more likely.

In some conditions the spleen becomes enormously enlarged and the slow circulation causes a disproportional amount of blood to be removed from the general circulation (splenic pooling). Gross splenomegaly is also accompanied by an increase in the plasma volume, so that although the total red cell mass may be normal, dilution by the increased plasma results in an apparent anaemia.

The white cells and platelets may also be affected by 'pooling' in the spleen or by premature removal from circulation. In addition there is evidence that the spleen may be one site of production of antibodies to red cells and platelets.

The part played by the spleen in immunity to infection is revealed by the increase in susceptibility to infection after removal of the spleen, particularly in infants and children. Such infections are often of a sudden and overwhelming nature and are in most cases due to bacteria. Splenectomy is avoided if possible in young children, but if it is considered essential prophylactic penicillin is prescribed to be taken regularly and continued at least until school-leaving age. Parents should be aware of the potential danger and make sure that the youngster takes the penicillin. They should also be prepared to get immediate medical advice at the first sign of any infection.

Blood Disorders

Some of the indications for removal of the spleen have already been discussed in previous chapters. When destruction of blood cells is excessive and shown to be due to overactivity of the spleen the operation can be a dramatic aid to treatment. It may be curative, as in cases of hereditary spherocytosis (see p. 58), or may be used to give relief of symptoms when the overactive spleen is part of another disease process as in some cases of lymphoma (see p. 135). If, however, other organs such as the liver are equally involved in cell destruction the benefit of splenectomy may be negligible.

In some cases of gross splenomegaly the sheer size and discomfort associated with it may warrant removal. The increased plasma volume and large mass of the organ may be a considerable strain on the heart and may also restrict breathing. In such cases, however, the possible benefit has to be weighed up very carefully against any possible adverse effects.

There is a curiously ill-defined condition called 'hypersplenism', in which one or more of the types of blood cells are reduced. It may be associated with splenomegaly where no underlying cause is found, or it may be secondary to a whole range of conditions associated with enlargement of the spleen. In some carefully selected patients the blood may return to normal following removal of the spleen.

The other indication for splenectomy, which has already been discussed, is in the process of staging for Hodgkin's disease (see p. 131).

Although a decision to remove the spleen may be made in many cases on the grounds of the history, clinical examination, and blood count, in some others more detailed investigations are required.

First, it is not always easy to distinguish between an enlarged spleen and other enlarged organs such as a kidney or tumour of the stomach or bowel. Special radiological investigations may supply an answer, but the most definitive

The spleen

method of identifying the spleen is to inject into a vein a small amount of red cells which have been labelled with a radioactive tracer and have also been damaged, for example by heat treatment, so that they will be removed rapidly from the circulation by splenic tissue. An external scanner will give a picture of the size and shape of the spleen.

The relative part played by the spleen and other organs such as the liver in destruction of cells may be assessed by labelling a sample of the patient's own red cells with a radioactive tracer and reinjecting them into the circulation. The fate of these cells is monitored by counting the radioactivity over both liver and spleen. If the radioactive cells are taken up mainly by the spleen splenectomy is likely to be of benefit, but if there is similar uptake in the liver, the operation is unlikely to be of help.

The operation of splenectomy is not always free from complications, the susceptibility to infections particularly in the very young, has already been mentioned. Another important hazard is a tendency to thrombotic lesions especially in the early postoperative period. This is at least partly associated with a rapid rise in platelets which usually occurs in the first couple of weeks. To prevent trouble patients are encouraged to be as active as possible after surgery.

If the operation has been technically difficult, because of adhesions to surrounding structures, there is a tendency for the base of the lung on the left side to be disturbed. Early physiotherapy helps to prevent this.

After splenectomy several characteristic changes are recognizable in the blood. Many of the red cells are fragmented or larger and flatter than normal (target cells), and they may contain inclusions or nuclear remnants (called Howell–Jolly bodies) which would normally be removed during passage through the spleen. These changes are described as those of hyposplenism.

In patients in whom splenectomy has failed to produce an

expected improvement, for example in those with haemolytic anaemia or thrombocytopenia, the presence of accessory splenic tissue may be suspected because of the lack of changes of hyposplenism in the blood.

18

Epilogue

In the foregoing chapters I have tried to give some idea of the wide spectrum of disorders of the blood, and the way in which knowledge about the mechanisms involved in these disorders has evolved over the last few decades. Fifty years ago some, but by no means all, of these conditions had been described, and in a few empirical treatment was available, but the underlying abnormalities were in most cases obscure.

In the past few years rapid advances in technology have revealed in ever-increasing detail the basic abnormalities leading to disorders of the blood. In some cases this has led to rational treatment, as in the megaloblastic anaemias. In others, as in the disorders due to congenital abnormalities of haemoglobin structure, the minute genetic changes which lead to profound disturbances of function have been revealed in detail, but as yet this knowledge can lead only to speculation as to whether at some future date it might be possible to correct the genetic defect. It is true that genetic counselling and ante-natal diagnosis are now, as a result of the basic research, being increasingly applied but therapeutic abortion is an emotive and debatable ethical subject, and a far from ideal way of preventing disease.

The remarkable developments in pharmacology in recent years have created their own problems, among them blood disorders related to drug sensitivity or immune reactions. On the other hand the damaging effect of a whole range of drugs on the growth of cells has been exploited in the management of the malignant blood disorders.

The ready communication between those studying particular blood disorders, and the pooling of their knowledge which is such a feature of modern medicine, has been of immense benefit in this field but it should be recognized that the major advances in treatment have been heavily dependent on the many thousands of patients who have participated in the studies made in specialized centres.

With progress in treatment have come new problems. Conditions which previously had a universally fatal outcome are now potentially curable, but the considerable dangers and complications along the way present those caring for patients with heavy responsibilities, anxieties and difficult decisions. Until we can learn more about the cause of the underlying malignant change further progress will probably be slow.

Research concerned with blood disorders, as in other fields, appears to go in phases — a rapid advance in one direction, and then a slowing down until the application of a new technique or the inspiration of an individual investigator causes a surge forward. One cannot predict what the future will hold any more than one could have imagined the present state of knowledge fifty years ago, but certainly understanding between patients and those who care for them must grow, to their mutual benefit.

Glossary

Agglutination: Clumping together of particles, such as red cells, produced by the reaction of a special type of antibody, called an agglutinin, which reacts with an antigen on the surface of the cells.

Agranulocytosis: Severe deficiency of the granulocytes.

Amniotic sac: The sac of fluid surrounding the fetus within the uterus.

Antigen: A substance which acts as a stimulus for the formation of an antibody.

Autoantibody: An antibody which reacts against a person's own cells.

Autoimmune disease: A condition in which antibodies are produced against components of the body's own tissues or their products.

Biopsy: Removal of a small piece of living tissue for microscopical examination.

Blast: Term used to denote a very early ancestral blood cell. Also applied as a suffix e.g. myeloblast, erythroblast.

Capillary: One of the mass of tiny blood vessels which forms a network in the tissues. Their walls are only one cell thick so oxygen, carbon dioxide and other substances can be easily exchanged between the blood and tissues.

-cyte: Suffix used to denote cell e.g. erythrocyte, meaning red cell.

Chelating agent: A chemical compound which forms complexes with metals.

Chemotherapy: Treatment with chemical compounds applied especially to treatment of malignant disease.

Chromosomes: Paired thread-like structures carrying the genes, that make up the nucleus of every cell. In humans

157

there are 23 pairs.

Clone: A group of cells arising from a single cell, and therefore having similar characteristics.

Duodenum: The first part of the small intestine into which the contents of the stomach empties; the bile and digestive juices from the pancreas are secreted into the duodenum.

Congenital: Dating from birth.

Cytoplasm: The cell substance which surrounds the nucleus.

Cytotoxic drug: One which damages or destroys cells.

Diverticulum: A sac or pouch developed at a point of weakness in the wall of the intestine.

Enzyme: A protein which increases the rate of a biological reaction without being used up itself.

Erythroblast: An immature red cell which still contains a nucleus.

Erythropoiesis: The production of red blood cells.

Erythropoietin: A hormone produced mainly by the kidney in response to reduced oxygen supply to the tissues; erythropoietin stimulates red cell production.

Ferritin: A soluble iron storage compound widely distributed in the various tissues of the body.

Gastric atrophy: A condition in which the specialised cells lining the stomach disappear, leading to loss of the normal secretions of the stomach.

Gastric parietal cell antibody: An antibody directed against the cells in the stomach which secrete acid.

Gastritis: Inflammation of the lining (mucous membrane) of the stomach.

Gene: The basic unit which transmits an hereditary factor and has a particular place on one of the chromosomes.

Gluten: A protein present in wheat and rye flour which is responsible for the elasticity of dough; coeliac disease is caused by a sensitivity to gluten.

Granulocyte: One of the group of mature white cells which have granules in their cytoplasm.

Haemoglobin: The red substance in red cells responsible for the uptake and release of oxygen.

Haemoglobinuria: The presence of haemoglobin in the urine.

Haemolysis: The breakdown of red cells with release of haemoglobin.

Haemopoiesis: The production of red and white cells and platelets.

Haemosiderin: An insoluble iron storage compound.

Haplotype: A group of genes so close together on a chromosome that they are inherited together.

Hormone: A substance secreted directly into the blood stream by one of the endocrine glands that has an influence on other organs or tissues.

Hypocellular: Reduced in cellularity.

Hypochromic: Deficient in haemoglobin.

Idiopathic: Of unknown cause.

Immunoglobulins: Proteins produced in response to the stimulus of a foreign substance and which act as antibodies.

Immunosuppressive drug: One which suppresses immune reactions.

Inherited: Passed on by genes from one generation to the next.

Jejunal biopsy: A small portion of the lining of the jejunum taken for microscopic examination.

Jejunum: The second part of the small intestine continuing on from the duodenum.

Laparotomy: Operation to open the abdomen.

Leucoerythroblastic anaemia: Anaemia characterized by the appearance of a few early white cells and nucleated red cells in the blood. It is an indication of bone marrow replacement by fibrous tissue or malignant cells.

Lymph node (or gland): Collection of lymphocytes enclosed in a fibrous capsule found at intervals along the course of the lymphatics.

Lymphoid tissue: Tissue, such as lymph nodes and spleen, which contains masses of lymphocytes.

Lymphoid: Belonging to the lymphocyte group of cells.

159

Blood Disorders

Molecular disease: A disease caused by a change in a single type of molecule.

Molecule: The smallest quantity of an element or compound which can exist while retaining its chemical characteristics.

Mucous membrane: The membrane lining various structures including the month, nose, stomach, gut and air passages.

Mutation: A change in the genetic material of a cell.

Myeloblast: The earliest recognizable granulocyte precursor; it is normally confined to the bone marrow.

Myeloid: Belonging to cells, other than lymphocytes, derived from bone marrow; particularly early granulocytes.

Myoglobin: An iron containing protein, similar to haemoglobin; which takes up oxygen into muscle fibres.

Neutropenia: A decrease in the numbers of neutrophil granulocytes in the blood.

Nucleus: The part of the cell which contains all the genetic material.

Pancreas: A gland which secretes digestive juices into the duodenum and also produces the hormone insulin.

Parietal cell: The cell in the lining of the upper part of the stomach which secretes acid.

Purpura: A rash caused by bleeding from small blood vessels in the skin.

Radioisotope: A form of an element which emits radiation.

Reticulocyte: A young red cell which still retains remnants of nuclear material, that appears like a fine network with special staining.

Reticulocytosis: An increase in the proportion of reticulocytes in the blood.

Sibling: A brother or sister.

Splenomegaly: Enlargement of the spleen.

Stem cell: The progenitor of all types of blood cells.

Telangiectasis: A small localized collection of distended capillaries which appears like a red spot.

Glossary

Thrombocytopenia: Reduction in platelets.

Thyroid: A large gland lying on each side of the windpipe at about the level of the Adam's apple; it secretes a hormone which regulates the metabolism of the body.

Index

Index

Index